Healing Touch
For Children

Healing Touch
For Children

Massage, reflexology and
acupressure for children

Mary Atkinson

First published in 2009 by Gaia Books

This edition published in 2017 by Albert Bridge Books

Contents

Foreword

In my role as Chief Executive of the Association of
Reflexologists, it is important to keep up to date with new
ideas, resources and research into the benefits of reflexology and other holistic therapies. So I was delighted to be
asked to write a foreword for *Healing Touch for Children*.
Mary Atkinson clearly wholeheartedly believes in the
therapeutic power of touch and her passion shines through
on every page of the book.

This inspiring book is written for parents wishing to
introduce the benefits of touch into the family home, but it
is also useful for therapists who are keen to encourage their
clients to support their own children through simple touch
techniques. It is informative and supportive, providing background information on each therapy, with a comprehensive
range of techniques and examples of when the techniques
should and should not be offered. The section on 'Treating
Common Ailments' provides a handy guide to childhood
well-being and offers gentle, natural solutions to be used in
conjunction with orthodox methods.

Touch therapy in the family home is simple, free and
extremely beneficial for both parent and child. The power
of touch can often be underestimated, but research over
recent years shows that sharing regular touch therapy with
a child can help increase self-esteem, boost concentration,

reduce pain, help bonding and bring the profound benefits of relaxation and a sense of calm in today's busy, challenging, high-tech world.

Our young people are so often bombarded from a tender age with physical and mental stresses, competitive pressures and high expectations from home, schools and peers. Positive touch through gentle massage and reflexology can help encourage children to discover a quiet and healing place within themselves that can help them cope better with the anxiety and stress that is leading to many health and behaviour problems today.

Indeed, as Mary Atkinson points out so clearly, sharing touch therapy can help teach children the essential life skill of conscious relaxation and an ability to react to stressful situations in a calm and rational. This self-awareness can lead to recognition of the warning signs of stress late in life.

Kerstin Uvnas-Moberg, a Swedish researcher and author of *The Oxytocin Factor, Tapping the Hormone of Calm, Love and Healing* believes that the feel-good effect of touch is linked with the release of oxytocin and other mood-enhancing chemicals during gentle touch therapy. Although research is still on-going, Kerstin suggests that this release of oxytocin is one of the reasons why touch has such a positive impact on countering the detrimental effects of stress and anxiety on our physical, emotional and mental health and well-being. And the good news is that oxytocin is released into the bodies of those giving as well as those receiving gentle touch so it can bring relaxation for parents too.

This book is a helpful reminder that simple touch can have profound benefits for both the giver and receiver. I would recommend it to therapists and parents alike.

Carolyn Story, Chief Executive, Association of Reflexologists

Introduction

Being a parent can be one of the most rewarding and enjoyable jobs in the world. Yet it is also one of the most demanding. As parents, the strains, pressures and competitive nature of modern living can make it almost impossible for us to have sufficient space in our day to take a step back and consider the most essential elements of happiness and well-being for our children – love, time and a nurturing touch. Children need to know they are special. Sometimes we do, quite literally, lose 'touch' with our children.

This book offers you the opportunity to re-establish the importance of sharing healing touch with your child. And the emphasis is on sharing. The routines and sequences described here are meant to be enjoyed *with* your child, rather than being viewed as an activity that you *do* to your child. Simply relax and let your own natural caring touch shine through – just five minutes a day can make all the difference. Invite your child to offer touch therapy to you, as well. Younger children, in particular, can be the world's best imitators and have wonderfully caring hands. Share the experience with grandparents and siblings, too – if the right occasion arises. You will be pleasantly surprised by the far-reaching physical and emotional benefits that this shared interaction can bring within the family.

How to use this book

The introduction to the book offers a basic explanation of why touch is so beneficial in the family home, especially in today's stressful world. It is not new information, but a valuable reminder of what parents have intuitively known for generations. The joy of touch is that it is simple, free and can be used just about anywhere, at any time, with the minimum of fuss and preparation. However, to ensure that you share a safe healing touch that offers maximum benefits for your child, it is wise to follow some basic guidelines – these are outlined in Chapter 1.

The next three chapters introduce specific touch therapies for children – head and shoulder massage, reflexology and acupressure – all of which complement each other. It is a good idea to read these sections and practise some of the techniques and suggested weekly routines on yourself or a willing adult before sharing them with your child. You'll find videos of the author demonstrating the techniques on the You Tube Channel - Positive Touch for Children with Mary Atkinson. Once you have learned the strokes, you can give your child some touch therapy whenever she needs it. Always remember that you do not need to be an expert to give a loving, caring massage or reflexology session; your child will take pleasure in your touch because it is yours.

Touch therapies can help ease minor childhood ailments such as headaches, constipation and sinus problems. Basic step-by-step sequences are illustrated in Chapter 5. Although not a substitute for medical advice or intervention, these gentle natural therapies offer a way of working with your child to overcome everyday health problems together. They do not diagnose or cure; they simply give a helping hand to your child's own natural healing resources. But do also enjoy sharing the benefits of nurturing touch when your child is feeling well, rather than simply using the routines to help ease the symptoms of minor ailments.

Finally Chapter 6 provides a self-help tool kit with routines that you can teach your child (or use yourself!) to gain relief from some of the common health conditions – such as tummy ache and leg cramp – that stop everyone enjoying life to the full from time to time. These techniques can be performed discreetly and are good for children to use when they are on the move.

The language of touch

Massage and touch therapy have been an integral part of family life for centuries in many Eastern cultures. For mothers in Asia, Eastern Europe and Africa, offering comforting touch to their babies and children is an intuitive maternal response – a way of connecting with them and communicating love, caring and respect. Once children reach the age of seven or eight, it feels perfectly natural for them to continue the tradition by offering massage to their parents and grandparents as a way of showing affection through their hands.

Pioneering studies

The importance of gentle touch from an early age was brought to the attention of Vimala McClure, founder of the International Association of Infant Massage, while she was working in a small orphanage in India in 1973. She came to realize that touch (not only from mothers, but from all care-givers) is one of the greatest gifts we can offer a child. Her pioneering work has shown how regular touch, which offers the gift of love and security, can be vital for a child's early growth and development. The benefits of caring touch from mothers, fathers and other carers continue past babyhood into adolescence and beyond. Studies under the direction of Tiffany Field at the Touch Research Institute in Miami show how touch can increase attentiveness in children, alleviate mild depression, reduce pain and boost the immune system. Gentle head and shoulder massage given to students prior to an exam has helped to relieve anxiety and slow down breathing. Other studies have shown how regular massage and reflexology can help with sleep patterns, hyperactivity and asthma.

For Mia Elmsater in Sweden and Sylvie Hetu in Canada, a profound belief in the vital importance of nurturing and respectful touch for children led them to set up the worldwide Massage in Schools Programme, with the vision of bringing clothed peer-massage into the school system.

The author of this book is co-founder, with Sandra Hooper, of an innovative Story Massage project which combines the therapeutic power of gentle massage with the creativity of story telling for children. Story Massage is now widely used in schools, special schools, hospices, hospitals and the family home.

Several studies show that five to ten minutes of massage every day can help boost concentration in children, and enable them to manage the activities of the day in a calmer way. One study showed that children tend to be less aggressive after regular massage, and another study demonstrated that children who offer massage to peers or parents show an improvement in motor skills.

Children deserve caring touch

Children can get just as stressed as adults – sometimes even more so. Our modern world is full of demands, choices and expectations, and children are bombarded with the noise of televisions, mobile phones and computers. They may also have worries about friendships, bullying, homework and disturbing items on the news. Then there is sibling rivalry, peer pressure, school attainment targets and concerns about their appearance.

Mental and physical health are directly linked to tension and stress. Sometimes the pressure on children builds up to such an extent that it manifests in a variety of different complaints, such as headaches, stomach upsets, mood changes and sleep disturbances.

For parents, it can be a real challenge to know the best way to guide and support children through the pressures and difficulties inherent in growing up in the 21st century. It is helpful to have an understanding of how stress affects your child's body and why it has such a profound and detrimental effect on health and well-being. With this knowledge, you can then devise your own ways of counterbalancing negative stress with positive relaxation and a regular caring touch.

Of course, not all stress is a bad thing. It can provide the motivation to finish tasks, give a competitive edge when playing sports and raise performance in exams. It also provides that wonderful tingling feeling before an exciting event. Stress only becomes harmful when it starts to affect someone's mental and physical health. It is a very personal reaction – everyone has a different stress threshold. What seems invigorating to one person at a certain time may cause anxiety to another person in a different situation. Too much stress for your child can build up over time and lead to mental, physical and emotional overload.

Fight or flight

In any stressful situation the body responds by releasing hormones, including adrenalin (also known as epinephrine), to prepare the body for instant action. This is known as the 'fight or flight' response and is a survival tactic designed to ensure that the body is at the peak of physical ability ready to fight an opponent, for example, or run from a burning building.

Muscles tense for optimum performance. The heart and lungs work extra hard to speed up the flow of blood and oxygen to the muscles and brain. Blood pressure and pulse rate rise. Breathing speeds up. The bladder and bowel empty to make the body as light at possible. Sweat glands produce more sweat to cool the body, ready for the expected physical threat.

The 'fight or flight' response worked perfectly in primitive times: once the body had discharged the increased energy supplies through fighting or fleeing, it relaxed and normal functions were restored. In modern times, however, although stress is often psychological, the body responds in the same way. Unless children have some outlet for the stress response – which, with an increasingly sedentary, screen-based lifestyle is often difficult – stress hormones may build up, causing them to live under a low level of 'crisis' for days, months or even years.

Redressing the balance

The accumulation in the body of stress hormones such as adrenalin and cortisol can exacerbate common childhood problems (both physical and emotional), including headaches, constipation, anxiety, niggling aches and pains, sleep problems, loss of confidence and lack of concentration. Stress hormones also depress the immune system, leading to greater susceptibility to diseases and allergies.

So how can parents redress the balance? Encouraging physical activity, a healthy diet, regular sleep and fresh air are all essential ways of counterbalancing stress. These healthy lifestyle patterns can be complemented by regular caring touch, which activates the parasympathetic nervous system and helps bring the body back into a state of calm and relaxation. Think how you instinctively hold a child's hand when he is afraid, or offer a gentle pat on the shoulder for reassurance. Touch encourages the release of a hormone called oxytocin, a natural antidote to stress.

The benefits of touch for your child

There is substantial research to show that touch therapy works on both a physical and psychological level to aid the emotional, physical and social health and development of children. Above all, it works on many different levels to offer closeness, security and comfort. It offers your child the chance to relax and let go in a safe environment, enabling her to recharge and refresh both mind and body away from today's frenetic lifestyle with its information and communication overload. In both the long and the short term, regular caring touch can:

● Target trouble-spots and help relieve localized tension, stiffness or aches, such as headache, eye strain and backache

- Encourage better-quality sleep, leading to an improved temperament
- Relax mind and body, easing tension and the cumulative effects of stress
- Teach children the essential life skill of conscious relaxation and an ability to react to stressful situations in a calm, rational way; self-awareness can lead to recognition of the early warning signs of stress later in life
- Offer individual attention, which enhances a child's awareness of being loved, valued, respected and safe; this in turn boosts self-worth and helps to create a positive body image and a feeling of ease with oneself
- Help prevent a build-up of impurities in the body, which can lead to muscle pain, headaches, skin disorders, sinus congestion and fatigue
- Increase lung capacity and encourage deeper, more regular breathing patterns
- Improve physical and mental energy levels, encouraging alertness, concentration and feelings of 'get up and go'
- Encourage a healthy immune system, helping to prevent and fight infections and allergies
- Promote the production of 'feel-good' hormones including oxytocin which helps to boost general well-being and bring a sense of calm and relaxation
- Help to calm aggressive or hyperactive behaviour
- Provide a valuable opportunity to share time together – laughing, having fun and using the imagination
- Build trust and intimacy through non-verbal communication, encouraging the release of any concerns that may have been bottled up and a chance to share confidences with your child in a calm, comforting atmosphere

- Take your child's mind away from any worries and doubts, enabling you to look at problems together from a different point of view and helping a child cope with daily pressures in a positive frame of mind
- Rekindle a bond with your child at times when your relationship is difficult, and provide emotional warmth and security to work through this stage together.

Chapter 1: Getting prepared

You can offer gentle, nurturing touch to your child in just about any situation. However, attention to minor details can often help make it a more enjoyable and rewarding experience for you both. It is well worth setting aside a few minutes to focus your thoughts and prepare yourself for sharing the benefits of touch.

Introducing your child to touch

Children who have enjoyed baby massage from a very early age tend to be familiar with touch and will respond well to the routines outlined in this book. However, those with little experience of regular touch will gain just as much benefit as those who have been massaged from birth. It may take a little more time for some children (especially older ones) to become accustomed to sharing respectful touch, but with patience and gentle persuasion at the right time, the chances are that you will soon find they start to relax under your gentle strokes – and ask for more. You should never force your child; healing touch is an experience to be enjoyed.

Children develop at different paces. Look at any group of children of the same age and you will notice that they are different sizes, shapes and temperaments, with different interests and approaches to life. You know your own child better than anyone else. You will know whether she is bursting with energy and constantly on the move, or whether she is full of questions or loves to reside in an imaginary world. And then these phases pass and new ones begin. Many of the suggestions offered in this book are guidelines – you will know which apply to you and your child at different stages in her development.

Time and place

Set time aside solely to be with your child, so that you can be fully focused on sharing safe touch together. Many children thrive on regular routine, so you may choose to use the same time and place each day or week. Others will prefer to have a massage or reflexology session on a more ad hoc basis. Younger children tend to have a short attention span, so try not to be over-ambitious. Aim for 10 to 15 minutes, but be aware that even two to five minutes can be a wonderfully rewarding experience.

Most children are better able to settle when they are not feeling tired or hungry. Massage or reflexology often works well as part of a bedtime routine, so try integrating some of the moves with a favourite bedtime story. Another popular time is after a bath, when it is natural to rub moisturizing oils into your child's skin. You can even massage younger children in the bath.

Touch therapy sessions can be great fun – use your sensitivity to plan the session in a way that you know will enhance your child's enjoyment. Try making up your own names for strokes, or encourage a younger child to follow the massage strokes on a favourite toy. Invite your child to smell some aromatic oils and choose her favourite one for the day. Use your imagination and get absorbed in creative play. There is no right or wrong way-just do what feels right for you and your child.

A safe touch

Touch therapies are only beneficial if they are given with care and respect for your child. Before you begin, it is advisable to be aware of a few simple safety guidelines, which will ensure that you both gain the maximum benefit from giving and receiving a massage.

Health cautions

Touch therapies are not substitutes for medical care and should not replace prescribed medication. Do not offer a session when you are feeling unwell, upset or rushed as you and your child may both end up feeling fraught and anxious.

Avoid massage, reflexology or acupressure if your child:
- Has an infection, rash or high temperature (especially if you are unaware of the cause)
- Has a contagious illness
- Is having a migraine attack
- Has been vaccinated in the previous week or is suffering from the after-effects of vaccination.

Seek advice from your doctor or specialist:
- If your child is under medical care for any on-going medical condition
- If you have any doubts about treating your child.

Avoid working over:
- Areas of recent injury, including sprains, strains, fractures and whiplash injuries
- Cuts, bruises, open wounds, areas of sunburn, bumps, bites and stings
- Athlete's foot, verrucas, warts.

Be aware of:
- Any skin allergies if using oils or creams.

Before a session

Always ask your child if she would like to receive a massage session from you today and respect her right to say 'no'. Sometimes children who love the experience of massage may not feel like it on certain days, so allow them the freedom to decline. If your child is reluctant at first, keep asking now and again; he may change his mind if he sees his siblings enjoying a massage.

Children can feel sensitive about their developing bodies. Make it clear from the outset that you will not touch any part of the body that your child does not wish to be touched. And ensure that you keep long hair tied back and that you remove any wristwatches, bracelets, large rings or dangling earrings. Also cover any cuts or abrasions on your hands.

During a session

Be aware that massage can release emotional tension and that you may find your child becomes tearful, angry or giggly. Stop if she feels faint or dizzy, or becomes distressed or uncomfortable in any way.

Offer plenty of positive encouragement as your child starts to relax with your touch. Make it clear that you are working together for her health and well-being. Invite your child to ask questions. Start to develop her natural curiosity in her own body and how she can look after her own health. Encourage your child to offer feedback on your strokes: invite her to say what she likes and dislikes, and to comment on the pressure and pace or whether she would like to stop altogether.

Be aware of your child's body language. Watch for squirming, wriggling or withdrawing. Younger children do not always have the words to express different sensations, so may simply say that something tickles or feels funny. If your child finds your touch ticklish, try giving a slower, slightly firmer massage and asking her to take some deep breaths to aid relaxation.

After a session

Encourage your child to sit quietly for a few minutes after the session to fully absorb the tranquil atmosphere – this may be the time when she feels ready to share any worries or concerns with you.

Avoid giving your child heavy meals after a full massage session; light snacks and fresh fruit are best. And she should drink plenty of water to speed up the elimination of toxins from her body. Leave any oils on the hair for a few hours. When washing them out, place a few drops of shampoo directly on the hair; do not wet the hair first, as this will cause a thin film of oil to remain on it, even after several washes.

Creating a healing space

You can offer massage and reflexology to your child just about anywhere and at any time of the day or night.

However, once you are both familiar with the moves, making a little effort to create a cosy, quiet atmosphere can turn it into a wonderfully calming and bonding experience for you both.

Peace and quiet

You will find it easier to relax if you are confident that you can enjoy time together without any distractions. Turn off the television and radio, and turn on the answer-phone. Check that any pets or other children are settled and safe. Your child might like to make a sign for the door to show that you do not want to be disturbed!

A cosy atmosphere

You may like to choose a favourite room for your session. Ideally it should be warm and free from draughts. Body temperature can drop during relaxation so have some blankets to hand. Natural daylight is most soothing to the eyes, or use side-lights or a dimmer switch. And consider music: quiet, soothing music can add a special touch. Most music shops now sell a selection of CDs to aid relaxation, and your child may like to be involved in choosing the music.

Oils and creams

All the sequences in this book can be done through light clothing, but you may prefer to use oil or cream. Using nourishing oils on the head and shoulders can help promote strong, healthy hair and soft, supple skin – although your child may not be willing to be persuaded! Similarly with aromatic oils: some children positively enjoy the scent, while others find it off-putting. If you do choose oils, follow the instructions carefully.

Hand care

Your hands are important. Do make sure they are clean, relaxed and warm, as cold hands can come as quite a shock to the system. Try to keep your nails trimmed and filed, to avoid scratching your child's skin.

Your own comfort

Depending on whether you are offering massage or reflexology, you will be in a different position. The comfort of your child is important, but so too is your own comfort. If you find yourself twisting or stretching, then you may end up feeling very tired or suffering aches and pains. Try to keep your back straight, but relaxed. Be aware of your posture and change position or alternate hands as necessary throughout the session. Choose clothes that enable you to move with ease – preferably something loose-fitting, short-sleeved and, if you are using oils, washable.

What you will need

Lay everything out, so that you have it ready before you start. Your child may enjoy helping with this, as part of the fun of the routine. You will need the following items:

- A chair or padded surface for your child to lie on
- A large and small towel
- Cushions or pillows for support
- Paper towels to wipe your hands on and to absorb any spillage
- Good-quality oil or cream (optional); place it on a washable surface, as oils can drip and stain
- Soft background music (optional)
- A clock (helpful to enable you to keep an eye on the time)

Inviting peaceful thoughts

There are several methods of relaxing and soothing both mind and body. Relaxation techniques and visualizations can be ideal ways of calming yourself before offering nurturing touch to your child. You can also use them with your child, speaking softly and changing the words to suit his age and interests. Older children may be able to use visualizations for themselves when they feel the need to ease away tension, focus their attention and quieten their busy minds.

Simple visualization

Practise this visualisation to experience the feeling of peace that it can bring. Stand with your feet shoulder-width apart or sit comfortably on an upright chair. Relax your knees and shoulders. Close your eyes if you feel comfortable with them closed.

Now imagine that you are a tree, and that your feet are like the roots of a great tree sinking deep down into the earth. Your body feels strong and stable, like the trunk of an ancient tree. Feel the connection with the ground beneath you. Imagine that branches of your tree are growing from your head and shoulders, reaching high into the blue sky above you. Picture the leaves of your tree opening into the sunlight and relaxing in the warmth and energy of the sun's rays. Feel the warmth. Enjoy the beauty of the blue sky. Be very quiet. Can you hear any birds singing?

Breathe in that feeling of natural warmth and relaxation. Allow it to spread through every part of you – from the top of your head to the very tips of your fingers and toes. Doesn't it feel wonderful? Now wriggle your fingers and your toes. Stay with this peaceful frame of mind.

Relaxation

Once you start to feel the difference between tense and relaxed muscles, you will instantly recognize when you are holding tension, and you can then make a conscious effort to relax and let go. This relaxation exercise, which you can enjoy doing on your own or with your child at any time of day (or night), involves deliberately tensing and relaxing different muscles in your body. You will find that it helps ease aches and pains, as well as relaxing both your mind and your body.

Sit or lie comfortably and loosen any tight clothing. Tense the muscles in your face. Make a very ugly face, with your eyes and mouth all screwed up. Hold this position for a count of five, then release. Repeat a second time. Now hunch your shoulders and then let them drop and relax. Feel the tension easing from your body.

Next, grip your fingers very tightly and then let go. This is a blissful feeling and can be repeated around other parts of the body. Perhaps your child could suggest which muscles to tense, hold and relax.

Choosing oils for massage

The massage routines illustrated in this book can all be performed through clothes, without the need for oils. However, there may be occasions when the use of oils can complement your massage.

Carrier oils

Carrier oils are natural vegetable oils that can be used as a lubricant to make massage flow more easily and bring the benefit of skin-to-skin contact. They are rich in vitamins, proteins and minerals to help moisturize, nourish and strengthen skin and hair, and may be mixed together if you wish. The most popular carrier oils for children are described here:

Coconut oil
Coconut oil is the perfect natural moisturizer for skin and hair. It is nourishing and soothing for dry skin conditions. Do always choose organic virgin coconut oil.

Sweet Almond oil
This oil is light and smooth to use. It helps protect and nourish the skin and is especially beneficial for dry, sensitive and irritated skin conditions. *Do not use sweet almond oil on anyone with a nut allergy.*

Sunflower oil
Organic cold-pressed sunflower oil is a safe, light oil that is suitable for all skin types, especially dry skin. It is nutritious because it contains high amounts of vitamins.

Essential oils
The tradition of mixing natural vegetable oils with aromatic essential oils for massage dates back centuries. You can buy oils and creams that are pre-blended with essential oils to help ease particular childhood ailments. Health-food stores, large supermarkets, major pharmacies and aromatherapy mail-order catalogues are good sources. Always check that any oils and creams are suitable for children. Alternatively you may like to make up your own blends to suit your child.

Pure essential oils are concentrated natural chemicals derived from different parts of a living plant, such as the flower, leaf or petal. They are non-greasy, volatile (meaning that they evaporate easily at normal temperatures) and characterized by an individual aroma. When used correctly, they can have a beneficial effect on mind, body and emotions. However, they are powerful substances and must be treated with caution. The therapeutic ingredients are inhaled and/or absorbed through the skin and into the bloodstream, where they travel around the body to fulfil their healing functions.

The following three pure essential oils are the most popular ones for children and are safe for home use, if applied as directed.

Lavender (*Lavandula angustifolia*)
A natural sedative, lavender induces calm and promotes restful sleep. It also has painkilling properties, so it is useful for easing headaches and alleviating muscular aches and pains, and helps to boost the immune system. Lavender is helpful in first aid for burns, stings, bites and bruises because it has antiseptic qualities that can assist the healing process.

Roman chamomile (*Anthemis nobilis*)
Beneficial for all stress-related conditions, Roman chamomile is a gentle oil with a soothing effect on mind and body. It can help lift anxieties and doubts and has a beneficial effect on skin disorders associated with emotional stress.

Mandarin (*Citrus reticulata*)
A mild, yet energizing oil with a mood-enhancing scent, mandarin can act as a mildly stimulating tonic, helping to

boost the circulation, and as a gentle sedative for reducing stress. It can also ease constipation, flatulence and digestive disorders. Do not use mandarin oil before going out in the sun because it may make the skin more sensitive to the sun's ultraviolet rays.

Safe use of essential oils

- Never apply essential oils undiluted (except lavender – one drop may be applied directly to superficial burns). For massage always dilute them with a carrier oil in the correct proportions.
- Do not take them internally. If essential oils are consumed accidentally, ask your child to drink a glass of milk and get immediate medical help. If oil gets into the eyes, rinse them with milk to ease the stinging. If in doubt, seek medical assistance.
- Buy essential oils from a reputable supplier and check any safety warnings on them. Avoid them if they are likely to cause irritation or aggravate a medical condition.
- Do not use pure essential oils during pregnancy, when breastfeeding or on babies, unless advised by a fully qualified aromatherapist.
- Store them in a cool, dark place away from children and pets.

Aromatherapy for children

Pure essential oils can be used in various ways. When mixing oils, be cautious about the amount of essential oil used. The recommended dose for children is one drop of essential oil to 5 ml (1 teaspoon) of carrier oil. *Do not add more essential oil.* Begin by measuring the carrier oil in a bottle or small container, then add the correct number of drops of essential oil. Stir gently with a spoon or cocktail stick, or roll the bottle in your hands to blend the oils.

You can make up a blend with 5 ml of carrier oil for each massage or bath, or you may prefer to make up 10 ml or 30 ml and store it in a bottle for future use. Suggested blends are described here and usually keep for a couple of months. Label bottles clearly with the ingredients and date, plus a warning that the oil is for external use only. Keep them well away from children and pets. Be aware that oils can stain, so be careful when using them, and place the container on a washable surface.

Suggested blends
Simple Massage and Bath Oil
10 ml carrier oil
2 drops lavender or mandarin or Roman chamomile
or
30 ml carrier oil
6 drops lavender or mandarin or Roman chamomile

Calming Bath
10 ml carrier oil
1 drop lavender
1 drop mandarin
or
30 ml carrier oil
4 drops lavender
2 drops mandarin

Comforting Bath
10 ml carrier oil
1 drop lavender

1 drop Roman chamomile
or
30 ml carrier oil
3 drops lavender
3 drops Roman chamomile

Reassuring Back Rub
10 ml carrier oil
1 drop Roman chamomile
1 drop mandarin
or
30 ml carrier oil
3 drops Roman chamomile
3 drops mandarin

Relaxing Foot or Hand Mix
10 ml carrier oil
1 drop lavender
1 drop Roman chamomile
or
30 ml carrier oil
4 drops lavender
2 drops Roman chamomile

Tummy Soothing Oil
10 ml carrier oil
1 drop mandarin
1 drop lavender
or
30 ml carrier oil
4 drops mandarin
2 drops lavender

Massage

Massage oil is best applied warm. Wash your hands, then rub them together or immerse them in a bowl of warm water for a few minutes. Place some carrier oil or massage blend in your palms and rub them together. Add more oil as necessary during the massage. Cover your child in a towel to keep her warm and ensure her privacy, and to avoid stains.

Baths

You can use natural vegetable oils as a lubricant in the bath, or dilute two to three drops of essential oil in 5 ml of carrier oil to add a therapeutic aroma. Fill the bath with water, then add the mixture and gently agitate the water before letting your child get in. Be cautious, as the bath surface may be slippery. Your child can play in the bath as usual. Essential oil bath blends are not generally recommended for children under the age of five.

Compresses

Compresses may be used hot or cold. A hot compress is good for cramps, chest congestion and muscular pain; a cold compress is best for headaches. Fill a bowl with 100 ml (3½ fl oz) of hot or cold water. Add one drop only of your chosen essential oil. Lay a facecloth or piece of clean cotton on the surface of the water to absorb the oil. Squeeze out any excess water and place the compress over the affected area. Reapply as often as necessary. This mix is usually sufficient for around four applications. *Always ensure the temperature is comfortable for your child.*

Inhalations

Essential oils can help with breathing, sleeping and calm-ing anxiety. If the problems arise at night, place one drop only of pure essential oil on the corner of the pillow, or the collar or back of your child's pyjamas. Allow the oil to dry before bedtime and keep well away from the child's eyes.

For older children, place one drop of essential oil on a paper tissue or cotton handkerchief. Wrap it in cling film or foil, and suggest that your child takes a sniff whenever he needs it. Do not use more than one drop of essential oil for inhalation.

Chapter 2 : Head and shoulder massage

Massage is a basic, nurturing instinct. We all use our natural healing power of touch in our everyday lives, often without realizing it. Once you have learned a few simple techniques, you will be able to develop your intuitive skills into a flowing sequence of movements and share a safe and beneficial head and shoulder massage with your child.

What is massage?

Massage is one of the oldest forms of healing. Throughout history, different cultures from all over the world have developed and used their own techniques to suit their needs. Today massage is enjoyed by people of all ages and all walks of life, with modern and ancient techniques being incorporated into routines to help relieve tension and stress and boost positive health and well-being.

Massage involves a series of movements with the hands, each of which are applied in a particular way to have a specific effect on the mind, body and soul. Brisk early-morning massage, for example, may awaken and refresh. Gentle massage in the evening can be the prelude to a deep, peaceful sleep. Similarly, massage can be applied in such a way as to either tone the muscles or relax them. As Hippocrates (c. 460–375 BCE), the 'Father of Medicine', wrote, 'rubbing can bind a joint that is too loose and also loosen a joint that is too tight'.

Therapeutic massage

Among the earliest records of therapeutic massage are those written in ancient Chinese books. The Chinese were particularly interested in studying the effects of pressure when applied to different parts of the body. Over time they developed techniques known as *amma*, using pressure at specific points to help the body heal itself. It was from these early discoveries that simple forms of acupuncture and acupressure were developed. In India, massage with aromatic oils and spices has long been an integral part of the ancient holistic system of Ayurvedic medicine.

In the West, the Greeks embraced massage as part of their health and fitness regimes, while the Romans enjoyed therapeutic massage at the end of their regular bathing routine. Records show that Julius Caesar was pinched all over every day to help relieve neuralgia, and Roman soldiers believed that massage helped them stay strong and fit during battle and aided recovery afterwards.

During the early 19th century a Swedish physiologist, Per Henrick Ling, introduced a system of exercises and massage movements that became known as physiotherapy, or physical therapy. During the First World War massage was used to provide pain relief and treatment for injured soldiers suffering from nerve damage and shell shock. Massage is now taken into homes, schools, offices, hospitals and even airports to help provide effective treatment for common ailments associated with our stressful modern lifestyles.

Introducing your child to massage

The massage moves included in this chapter concentrate on the shoulders, arms, back, head and face. These are areas where we all tend to hold a lot of tension, so massage can bring children almost instant calming benefits; they are also easily accessible, and touching them is unlikely to cause any embarrassment.

Some children love to be massaged, while others may be a little apprehensive at first. When you are both in the mood for massage, start with a gentle rub of the shoulders or by 'shampooing' the hair, then introduce a few new moves when your child asks for more. Keep the pressure fairly light and work at a rhythmic speed. In general, slower movements are more relaxing, while brisker movements are more invigorating. Avoid massaging over your child's spine or any really bony protrusions. And be extra gentle on the face.

Massage positions

Choose a position that is comfortable for you both. Make every effort to ensure that your child feels warm and secure. Be aware of your own posture to avoid any aches and pains. Depending on the size of your child, you might like to try the following:

- Your child sits on a chair or stool (but do choose one that does not squeak or wobble). You stand or sit behind your child to offer the massage. Experiment with different chairs and cushions to ensure that you are both at the right height.

- You sit on the floor or on a bed, with your back resting against the wall or bedhead. Prop yourself up with pillows for comfort. Your child sits between your outstretched legs, with her head against your chest. You may like to support her back with a small cushion or rolled-up towel. An alternative is sitting with your child on your knees facing forwards.
- Your child lies on a bed, the floor or a table. You kneel, sit or stand by her side, depending on the height. Use plenty of padding to make the surface comfortable, and cover your child with a towel, especially if you are using oils.

Basic massage techniques

The massage sequences in this book are based on several simple techniques that are performed in a specific way to have a beneficial effect on mind and body. Try experimenting with the different moves and various levels of pressure and speed. You will soon find those that your child enjoys most. Some of the techniques may feel a little awkward at first, but remember that it is your intention that really matters. Apply each stroke with the care and affection that your child deserves and you will both feel uplifted and refreshed by the shared experience of massage.

The massage moves can be performed through light clothing or using oils direct on the body. You can find out more about using oils in Chapter 1. You'll find videos of the author demonstrating the techniques on the You Tube Channel - Positive Touch for Children with Mary Atkinson.

Holding

A comforting hold is the perfect way to start and end a massage. Holding gives both you and your child the opportunity to slow down and focus your minds. Use the whole surface of your palms and fingers to gain optimum contact. The warmth generated by your hands can add to the relaxing effect on your child. For extra benefit, try adding a little pressure to your hold.

Stroking

Stroking is usually a favourite with children. Keep your hands and fingers supple and slightly cupped, so that they naturally mould to the contours of your child's body. Glide them smoothly over the area, using a gentle pressure initially and then gradually increasing it to suit your child's preferences. This soothing, rhythmic stroke helps prepare the body for deeper massage. You can perform it in straight sweeps or in a large or small circular movement. You can stroke with one hand, with both hands together or with the soft pads of fingers or thumbs.

Rubbing

Brisk rubbing has a wonderfully warming effect and can help relax and revive both mind and body. Keep your wrists flexible, with your fingers held quite straight. Rub over the surface of your child's skin using short, invigorating movements, back and forth in a sawing motion in any direction. You can use the palms or heels of your hands, the pads of several fingers or even a loosely clenched fist.

Kneading

Once an area of the body is warmed by stoking or rubbing then you can use kneading to help stretch and relax tight and tired muscles. As the name suggests, the technique is rather like kneading bread dough and involves grasping and lifting a fleshy area of muscle, then pressing, squeezing or rolling it before releasing. Depending on the size of the area, you can use one or both hands or your fingers or thumbs. Check the pressure carefully with your child.

Tapping

These three brisk, energizing strokes are fun to give as well as receive. The three variations all include striking or tapping the skin and then releasing it in a rapid, rhythmic way. Your hands bounce back up as soon as they land. Start with a light pressure and gradually increase it to a level that feels good for your child. Work around any especially bony areas and always avoid the spine. Allow your hands to move around rapidly to cover the whole area.

Beating

Make your hands into loose fists. Use the sides of your fists or the backs of loosely clenched fingers and the heels of your hands. Use both hands alternately to strike the flesh gently in a rhythmic way. Do not work over the spine.

Patting

Use the palms or backs of your hands to tap the skin gently with a light, springy movement. Use both hands simultaneously or alternately, slowly or more quickly, maintaining a steady rhythm.

Tabla

This move is named after northern Indian tabla drums, which are played with the pads of the fingers. Lightly and briskly drum your fingers in a rhythmic movement – there is no need for your fingers to tap in any particular order. Tabla feels rather like raindrops.

Basic massage sequence

This series of movements takes around seven to ten minutes to perform and includes varying combinations of gentle, soothing strokes and brisk, stimulating moves. Adapt the routine as you wish, spending longer on favourite strokes or omitting others to suit your child. Let her know what to expect and invite her to ask any questions before you begin and during the massage.

Head, shoulder and back massage

This routine is designed to be carried out with your child in a sitting position, but you can adapt this if she prefers to lie down. Do ensure that your child is well supported so that she can relax fully and even sleep during the massage if she wishes.

1. First hold

Rest your hands, palms downward, on your child's shoulders. Hold for a count of three. Invite your child to take three deep breaths, in and out.

2. Back circles

Place your hands on your child's upper back, one on either side of the spine. With fingers pointing upward, stroke your hands up and around the shoulder blades, tracing generous circles. Keep the movement slow and smooth, with more pressure on the upward movement. Repeat three times.

3. Back rubbing

Place one hand across your child's upper chest to offer support. With the flat of the other hand, rub across the upper back, the tops of the shoulders and upper arms in small zigzag movements. Rub briskly, covering the whole area. To add some variety, you can also use the heel of your hand or rub with small, circular movements.

4. Shoulder kneading

With your hands resting on your child's shoulders, gently knead the soft flesh beneath them between your palms and fingers. Feel for the tension that so often creeps into these hard-working muscles. Press, lift, squeeze and release in a rhythmic action, like kneading bread dough. Be careful not to press too hard or too suddenly – be aware of your child's body language. Afterwards gently stroke and soothe the area.

5. Beating on the upper back

Now for some stimulating action: place your hands in loosely clenched fists and gently beat the upper back and top of the shoulders. Use both hands alternately, so one works after the other. Avoid any bony prominences.

6. Back stroking

Starting on the right shoulder, stroke with the palm of one hand to midway down the back. Now repeat the stroke with the other hand. As one hand finishes, the other begins. Work across the back with this wave-like stroking movement.

7. Arm tapping

Using the flat of your hands, gently tap from the top of the shoulders all the way down to your child's hands and back up again. Use both hands alternately. Repeat.

8. Arm kneading

With your hands on the top of each arm of your child, gently squeeze, release and hold. Move your hands a little further down the arms and repeat the squeezing and holding movement. Work all the way down to the elbows and back up to the tops of the arms.

9. Shoulder stroking

Bring your hands to the base of your child's neck and stroke along the top of the shoulders and down the upper arm to the elbow. Release the pressure and glide gently back to the starting position. Repeat three times.

10. Neck rubbing

Support your child's forehead with one hand. With the flat of two or three fingers of the other hand, rub lightly and briskly around the back of the neck and under the base of the skull.

11 Head rubbing

Rest your hands lightly on your child's head. Using the flat of one hand, gently rub over the scalp, working from the front of the head to the back. You may choose to support your child's head while rubbing with the other hand.

12. Hair 'shampooing'

Place your hands in a claw-like position on top of the head and use the fleshy pads of your fingers and thumbs to make small circular 'shampooing' movements all over the scalp. Maintain an even pressure, moving all round the scalp and feeling it move beneath your fingers.

13. Tabla on the head
Gently drum the pads of your fingers in a random fashion all over the top of your child's head. Continue this light and bouncy tabla movement over the top of the shoulders and neck.

14. Head and shoulder stroking
Stroke both hands from the top of the head downwards, over your child's shoulders and upper back, in a long, sweeping movement. Release, then bring your hands back to the top of the head and repeat several times. Ask whether your child prefers the move to cover his ears or fall behind them.

15. Temple circles
Place the flat of your hands over your child's temples, with your fingers facing away from you. Make slow, circular movements over the area. Repeat three to four times.

16. Forehead stroking
Gently stroke your child's forehead using the palms of your hands. Stroke upwards or across the forehead from one side to the other. Keep the movement soft and flowing.

17. Final hold
Finish by gently resting your hands on the top of your child's head for a count of five. Smooth your child's hair back into place.

Checklist

Use this list of moves as a prompt so you do not need to interrupt the flow and enjoyment of the massage by turning the pages of the book.

- First hold
- Back circles
- Back rubbing
- Shoulder kneading
- Beating on the upper back
- Back stroking
- Arm tapping
- Arm kneading
- Shoulder stroking
- Neck rubbing
- Head rubbing
- Head 'shampooing'
- Tabla on the head
- Head and shoulder stroking
- Temple circles
- Forehead stroking
- Final hold

Chapter 3: Reflexology

Offering caring touch to your child's feet through some simple reflexology techniques can bring a surprising number of far-reaching benefits to you and your child. This ancient art, which has been rediscovered and developed as a valuable complementary therapy in recent years, is based on the same guiding principle as massage – the healing power of touch.

What is reflexology?

Reflexology works by applying finger and thumb pressure to the feet and hands to help promote and maintain health and well-being. This natural therapy is based on the principle that specific points, known as reflex points, in the feet and hands relate to the different organs, functions and parts of the body. A full reflexology treatment involves working all the reflex points, but specific points can also be used for 'self-help' and 'first-aid' measures.

The art of reflexology has been known to humans for thousands of years. Records show that it was practised by the early Japanese, Chinese and Egyptian civilizations. A pictogram (or pictorial symbol) in the Physician's Tomb at Saqqara in Egypt, dating back to 2300 BCE, depicts people giving and receiving hand and foot therapy.

Zone therapy

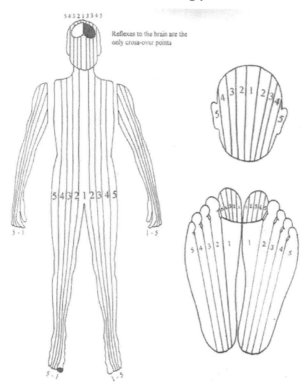

Reflexes to the brain are the only cross-over points

The 10 Zones of the body

Reflexology is based on the theory that the body is divided into ten channels, or zones. These zones extend from each toe, up through the body to the head and down the arms to the hands, and back again. Within each zone there is a flow of energy that affects all parts of the body within the same zone. Periods of illness, stress or injury – however minor – can cause blockages in these vital energy pathways, thereby upsetting the body's natural equilibrium. At the beginning of the 20th century the American surgeon Dr William Fitzgerald discovered that by applying pressure generally to the zones on the feet and hands it is possible to help clear any imbalances and relieve pain in other areas within the same zone; this was the start of zone therapy.

Zone therapy was further developed by American physiotherapist Eunice Ingham, often considered the pioneer of modern reflexology. She developed charts that show the exact location of reflex points and areas relating to specific organs and parts of the body. These charts have been developed over the years. The right foot corresponds to the right side of the body, and the left foot to the left side. Some parts of the body are found only on one side and are therefore represented only on one foot.

Visualizing the reflexes

To help work out the position of the reflexes on the feet, try to visualize horizontal lines running across each foot. The toes reflect your child's head area, with the upper part of the foot reflecting your child's chest and upper back. The arch of the foot represents your child's abdomen and middle back, above and below the waist. The heels of the feet represent your child's hip area and lower back.

The foot maps on the next page show the location of different reflexes for your interest. The sequences in this book only work on reflex points that are appropriate for children and some are not included in these foot maps. You'll find videos of the author demonstrating the techniques on the You Tube Channel - Positive Touch for Children with Mary Atkinson.

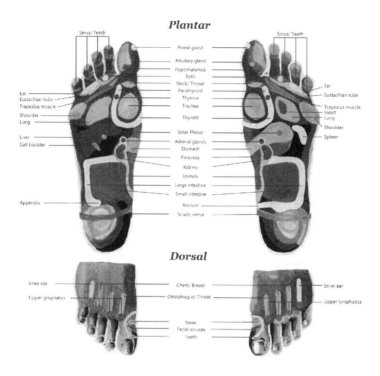

Plantar

Sinus/ Teeth

Pineal gland
Pituitary gland
Hypothalamus
Eyes
Neck/ Throat
Parathyroid
Thymus
Trachea
Thyroid

Solar Plexus
Adrenal glands
Stomach
Pancreas
Kidney
Ureters
Large intestine
Small intestine

Rectum
Sciatic nerve

Ear
Eustachian tube
Trapezius muscle
Shoulder
Lung

Liver
Gall bladder

Appendix

Ear
Eustachian tube
Trapezius muscle
Heart
Lung
Shoulder

Spleen

Dorsal

Inner ear

Upper lymphatics

Chest/ Breast
Oesophagus/ Throat

Nose
Facial sinuses
Teeth

Inner ear

Upper lymphatics

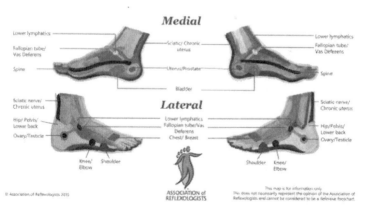

Medial

Lower lymphatics

Fallopian tube/
Vas Deferens

Spine

Sciatic/ Chronic
uterus

Uterus/Prostate

Bladder

Lower lymphatics

Fallopian tube/
Vas Deferens

Spine

Sciatic nerve/
Chronic uterus

Hip/ Pelvis/
Lower back

Ovary/Testicle

Lateral

Lower lymphatics
Fallopian tube/Vas
Deferens
Chest/ Breast

Knees/
Elbow

Shoulder

Shoulder

Knees/
Elbow

Sciatic nerve/
Chronic uterus

Hip/Pelvis/
Lower back

Ovary/Testicle

© Association of Reflexologists 2015

ASSOCIATION of
REFLEXOLOGISTS

This map is for information only.
This does not necessarily represent the opinion of the Association of
Reflexologists and cannot be considered to be a definitive footchart.

Foot Maps

Introducing your child
to reflexology

Some children love to have their feet touched, while others are less enthusiastic – and this can change with age. You know your own child best. Reflexology is a wonderfully relaxing pleasure to be enjoyed, but don't force it. Make it a game: let your child fidget and move and ask lots of questions. As your child gets older, she may well become fascinated with the way that different reflexes relate to different parts of her body. Spend some time explaining this, and invite her to work on your feet too.

Practising the techniques

Begin with a gentle rub of the feet to get your child used to the feel, then slowly progress at your child's pace. You can do reflexology anywhere (you do not even need to remove the socks), so take the opportunity to rub or press on a few reflex points when you are sitting together on the sofa, playing on the floor or when your child is in bed. Just a couple of minutes can make all the difference. If you find that your child asks for more, start to set aside a regular time for reflexology.

With practice, you will soon master the reflexology techniques and will become more sensitive to the 'feel' of the reflexes beneath your fingers and thumbs. Your child may experience a fleeting sensation – such as slight discomfort, sharpness or a twinge – when certain reflexes are touched. This indicates that these reflex areas need a little extra attention. By encouraging feedback from your child, you can work together to make each session as effective as possible.

Feet or hands?

Feet are more sensitive to the touch than hands. The soles of the feet contain around 70,000 nerve endings, making them among the most sensitive parts of the body. Reflexology can affect these sensory nerve endings, helping the body to relax and rebalance itself. So it is preferable for you to work on your child's feet, while encouraging her to work on her hands for self-help.

Reflexology positions

Spend a little time making sure that you are both comfortable and well supported. You should be able to move freely and have access to both your child's feet without stretching or twisting. Ensure that you can see her face to check for any signs of discomfort, so that you can stop the session or adjust your pressure. Your child may like to cover herself with a special blanket or surround herself with favourite toys. Some different reflexology positions are described here:

- Your child lies on a bed or reclining chair. You sit on a lower chair or stool, facing her feet. Use extra pillows to prop her up, if this is more comfortable. Ensure that her feet are at the bottom on the bed, so that you can reach them without stretching. You need to be able to work on the underside of the foot with comfort.
- Your child sits on a chair with her legs resting on a stool or small table of similar height. Alternatively, he rests his feet on your lap, on top of a cushion. You sit facing him on a stool, chair or cushion that enables you to maintain a good posture.

- Your child rests on a pile of cushions on the floor. You kneel or sit cross-legged, or with your legs outstretched, on the floor with your back against a wall or a heavy piece of furniture. Your child's feet and legs can rest on a cushion on your lap or on the floor, whichever is most comfortable.

Simple reflexology techniques

The reflexology sequences in this book are founded on a few basic techniques that are used to work the reflex areas of the feet and hands. Different techniques are used, depending on the size and location of the reflex area. Experiment with the various types of movement to find which one is best for you and your child. It is important to get the pressure right – so keep asking for feedback. Keep your touch gentle, but firm enough to avoid tickling. Watch your child's facial expressions for any signs of discomfort.

You do not need to use any medium for working on the feet. If you choose to use an oil or cream, be frugal – too much can cause your hands to slip and slide over the skin.

Supporting the foot

When applying reflexology it is important that your hands work together. One hand is used to support and steady the foot, enabling the other hand to reach and work the reflex areas effectively. Keep your supporting hand as relaxed as possible. Change hands and positions to help you contact the different areas comfortably.

Caterpillar walk

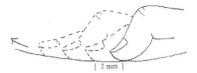

THUMB WALK OR "CATERPILLAR WALK"
BEND AND STRAIGHTEN THE FIRST JOINT OF
THE THUMB, GRADUALLY CREEPING FORWARD

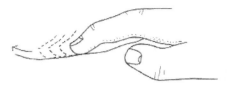

THE SAME MOVEMENT IS USED FOR FINGER WALKING

Caterpillar walking with your thumb is one of the most common techniques in reflexology. Practise on your own arms or hands. Begin by placing your right thumb on your left arm or hand. Now bend your thumb at the first joint, the one nearest to the nail. Slightly unbend and then bend your thumb so that it creeps forward in tiny steps. It is not a pushing action – more like a caterpillar walking.

As you take each tiny step, let the outer padded edge of your thumb press down, then release. Keep the pressure constant and even, with the thumb bent and in contact with the skin at all times. Move your thumb in a forward direction. You can work with your right or left thumb, whichever you find most comfortable. At first you may find that your thumb is taking large steps, but with practice they will get smaller and more precise.

Fingers can also do the caterpillar walk. They exert less pressure than the thumbs, so for some bony areas (such as the top of the foot) use one of your fingers – usually the index finger. The aim is to bend the finger it at the first joint, nearest the nail, and take small steps, edging forward and keeping the rest of the finger as straight as possible. The most common mistakes are bending your finger too much or pushing down too hard with your fingertips. It may take a little time to master the technique, so keep practising and remember that it is your caring touch that matters most.

Thumb and finger glides

You can also try gliding your thumb or fingers over the reflex points. Exert a gentle, even pressure as you slide the padded area of your thumb or fingers over the skin. There are times when these glides are easier to manage than caterpillar walking, both for you and your child, and they make a useful addition to your reflexology tool kit.

Static pressure

For very small areas, especially on little feet, you may find it easier simply to use the padded area of your thumb or finger to apply pressure on a reflex point and then release. Do be careful not to contact the skin with your nails, as this can be painful.

Circular pressure

An alternative to simple point pressure is to apply a static, circular pressure with the padded area of your thumb or finger, clockwise on a reflex point. Make the movement slow and deliberate. Keep your child's foot well supported with your other hand.

Zone walking

This is a useful technique to cover all the main reflexes in a short space of time and encourage the free flow of energy through the body. With your child's foot well supported, use a thumb or finger to 'walk' or glide through each zone from the heel to the toe on the underside of the foot.

Start at Zone 1 on the right foot. Walk or glide up from the heel to the big toe, then release. Now repeat this in Zones 2, 3, 4 and 5 on the right foot, then also on the left foot. Use this as a mini reflexology treatment or at the start of any of the reflexology sequences featured in this book.

Basic reflexology sequence

If your child enjoys reflexology, then this simple seven-to ten-minute sequence is the perfect way to encourage her own healing mechanisms to boost good health and prevent ill health. Do make sure you are both comfortable. You may need to change hands and positions throughout the sequence – do whatever feels best for you and your child. Try doing this routine once a week.

Relaxing the feet

Start your reflexology session by relaxing your child's feet. These moves will help your child become calmer and more receptive.

1. Reassuring hold

Cradle your child's heels in the palms of your hands. Hold for a few seconds.

2. Nurturing strokes

With one hand supporting the foot, use the other to stroke down the instep of the right foot with the palm of the hand. Repeat several times. Repeat on the left foot. These flowing strokes help warm and prepare your child's feet for massage and reflexology.

3. Rocking movements

Gentle 'back and forth' movements can help ease any tension and loosen your child's feet. Sandwich your child's right foot between your palms. Keeping your hands soft, move the flat of your hands gently backward and forward across the top and bottom of the foot to create a rocking sensation. Repeat on the left foot.

4. Kneading

Start with your hands cradling your child's right foot, fingers on top of the foot and thumbs on the underside. Now gently massage the soles of the foot with the fleshy pads of your thumbs. Move your thumbs in circles, using a gentle, even pressure to cover the sole. Repeat on the left foot.

5. Rotations

With your child's foot well supported with one hand, use the other to gently grasp the big toe between the thumb and fingers. Rotate the toe three times in one direction, then three times in the reverse direction. Continue with the other toes if you wish. This move has a surprisingly relaxing effect. Move your elbows out to the sides to do it more effectively.

6. Diaphragm rocking

The diaphragm line follows the lower edge of the ball of the foot, running from one side to the other. If you bend the toes towards the underside of the foot, you will see the natural crease that is formed. There is also a natural colour change where the ball of the foot meets the arch. This is the diaphragm line.

Gentle rocking movements along the line can have a wonderfully restful and reassuring effect. With one hand grasping your child's toes, place the thumb of your other hand on the diaphragm line on the outside edge of the foot. As you gently press in, bend the toes and carefully rock them forward. Release the pressure and gently rock them back. Move your thumb a little further along the diaphragm line and repeat the toe rocking. Repeat until your thumb reaches the inner edge of the diaphragm line. This technique can be used on its own or incorporated into any of the reflexology sessions in the book.

7. Solar plexus soothing

Pressing on the solar plexus reflex points (which are found in the hollows in the centre of the diaphragm line on both feet) can have a calming effect on the whole body. This technique forms an integral part of many reflexology routines for common ailments. Press the pads of your thumbs on the solar plexus points on both feet. Hold for a count of three, then release the pressure. Repeat three times. For added benefits, incorporate a breathing exercise while working on the points. Keep your child's feet well supported at all times. Suggest that your child takes a deep, relaxing breath in as you press on the points, then breathes out as you release your pressure. This makes an excellent way of starting and finishing your reflexology routines, or it can be beneficial on its own.

Working the reflexes

Once your child's feet are warm and relaxed, you can begin working on the reflexes. Start with your child's right foot, then repeat the sequence on the left foot, with an awareness that certain reflexes appear only on the right or left foot. Always use one hand to support the foot that you are working on. Change hands whenever feels right for you. The reflexes in this sequence are found mostly on the underside of the foot.

1. Head
Location: the padded area of the big toe on the underside of the foot.

Technique: with one hand keeping your child's big toe steady, use your other thumb to 'walk' or stroke, covering the whole of the padded area.

2. Brain
Location: top of the first three toes, just behind the nails.

Technique: starting with your child's big toe, use your thumb to press on the top of the big toe. Hold for a count of three. Do the same on the next two toes. Keep the foot well supported. You may find that it helps to place your hand in a fist beneath your child's toes.

3. Neck and throat
Location: base of the big toe, on the underside, top and sides of the toe.

Technique: with one hand supporting your child's foot, use your other thumb to 'walk' or glide all around the base of the big toe. Reposition your hands as necessary. Repeat.

4. Sinuses

Location: backs and sides of all five toes.

Technique: depending on the size of your child's toes, use your thumb or fingers to 'walk', glide or squeeze up the backs and sides of the big toe, starting at the base and working upwards. Repeat on each toe in turn. Reposition your hands as necessary.

5. Eyes

Location: on the ball of the foot, under the first bend of the second toe.

Technique: with the fingers of your supporting hand keeping the upper part of your child's foot steady, use your working thumb to press on the reflex point. Hold for a count of three, or make three circular pressure movements in a clockwise direction.

6. Ears

Location: on the ball of the foot, under the first bend of the little toe.

Technique: use the same technique as for the eye reflexes above.

7. Spine

Location: along the inside edge of the foot.

Technique: use your supporting hand to move your child's foot so that your working thumb can reach the area comfortably. You may find that it helps to place one hand in a fist on the sole of the foot to offer extra support. Starting at the inner edge of the big toe, use the thumb of your other hand to 'walk' down the edge of the foot, always moving in a forward direction following the natural curve of the foot. Change hands and 'walk' back to the big toe.

8. Lungs

Location: the large, padded area known as the ball of the foot.

Technique: use your thumb to 'walk' over whole area. You can work from the diaphragm line upwards, or across the foot, as you wish. Keep the foot well supported with your other hand.

9. Diaphragm

Location: a line that follows the lower edge of the ball of the foot, running from one side to the other. If you bend the toes towards the underside of the foot, you will see the natural crease that is formed. There is also a natural colour change where the ball of the foot meets the arch. This is the diaphragm line

Technique: use your thumb to 'walk' or glide along the line, working from one side of the foot to the other, then back again. Keep the foot well supported with your other hand.

10. Liver and gall bladder

Location: beneath the ball of the foot, mainly on the right foot.

Technique: use your thumb to 'walk' or glide over the area, working from the outer edge of the foot to the inner. Change hands and work in the opposite direction. Alternate hands as necessary. Keep the foot well supported.

11. Small and large intestine

Location: in the middle of the sole of the foot. The large intestine (colon) continues from the right foot to the left foot. The lower edge of the colon covers the top of the heel on the left foot.

Technique: With one hand supporting the heel of the foot, use the thumb of your working hand to 'walk' or glide over the area, working from the outer edge of the right foot across to the inner edge. When working on the left foot start by working this area from the inner edge to the outer edge. Change hands and work in the opposite direction.

12. Bladder

Location: the soft puffy area on the inside of the foot.

Technique: use your thumb or finger to 'walk' or glide over the bladder reflex and up towards the kidney reflex positioned in the arch of the foot in line with the big toe. If this area is not well defined on your child's foot, 'walk' or glide across the middle of the sole of the foot. Keep the foot well supported with your other hand.

13. Adrenal gland

Location: above the kidney reflex, which lies beneath the diaphragm line, in line with the big toe.

Technique: With one hand supporting the foot use the thumb of your working hand to press on this reflex. Hold for a count of three, then release. Use a light touch, as it can be sensitive.

Working the left foot

Now repeat the rest of the sequence on the left foot, including the spleen reflex after Step 9. If time permits, you may choose to end with solar plexus soothing.

14. Spleen

Location: beneath the ball of the foot on the outer edge of the foot in line with the fourth and little toe, *on the left foot only.*

Technique: use your thumb to 'walk' or glide over the area.

Chapter 4: Acupressure

This ancient form of Chinese medicine is becoming increasingly popular as a natural form of healthcare for all the family. Based on working on specific points to influence the flow of subtle energies through the body, acupressure can offer an effective way of helping to alleviate the symptoms of many common ailments and promoting positive health and well-being in your child.

What is acupressure?

Acupressure is a branch of traditional Chinese medicine dating back thousands of years. It is similar to acupuncture – but without the needles. It involves applying pressure (usually with the fingertips, thumbs or elbows) to points on the body. Although it is no substitute for a full treatment from a trained practitioner, working on specific points can help to relieve your child's minor ailments. Acupressure also offers a valuable self-help tool for both you and your child.

Qi and the meridians

Acupressure is based on the theory that Qi energy (pronounced chee, and also spelt Chi) flows along a network of invisible channels, known as meridians, which link all parts and functions of the body so that it works as an integrated unit. Twelve main meridians have been identified, each with a specific function and relating to a specific organ in the body, such as the liver, gall bladder and spleen. Some of the meridians are linked to the relaxation of mind and body, while others are linked to the stimulation of mind and body.

If the flow of Qi along a meridian is blocked or weak, or overactive, this may give rise to ill health. Applying pressure to specific points – which may not even be near the problem area – stimulates and rebalances the flow of Qi, thus boosting the body's natural healing powers and promoting health. Acupressure points each have a precise location and therapeutic effect on the mind and body. For ease of reference for practitioners, they are named after the meridian on which they lie and their exact location on it. These abbreviations are used in this book.

We are all unique

With acupressure, as with other holistic therapies, we are all considered unique and the main aim of treatment from a trained practitioner is to restore the balance of physical, emotional and spiritual aspects of each individual. As we are all so different, the sensations experienced and response to working the acupressure points will not be the same for everyone. Do work closely with your child to discover what feels comfortable and supportive for him as an individual.

Safety points

Follow these simple guidelines to ensure safe use of acupressure:

- Do not use these acupressure points on yourself, or anyone else, when you are pregnant or breastfeeding, if

you have high blood pressure or you have been drinking alcohol
- Do not apply acupressure directly to wounds, bruises,
or veins; always work around these areas
- Stop if you or your child feels ill or uncomfortable.

Locating acupressure points

Acupressure points tend to be positioned in small depres-
sions or hollows in the body structure. Generally, corre-
sponding points are found on either side of the body. You
may need to spend a little time finding the exact spot, as
these can vary from person to person. Follow the location guidelines given for each point, then use the tip of a
finger to explore the area. You will know when you have
found the point because, when it is pressed, your child
will often feel a slight tingling or heightened sensitivity,
which passes as you apply pressure.

For some of the points mentioned, you need to find
the location using the width of the fingers – this means
the fingers of the person being treated, so you may need
to enlist your child's help to find the right spot. Children
are often fascinated by this new way of discovering more
about their own bodies and are usually willing to help.

When locating the points and working on them, use
the soft pads on your fingers and thumbs to avoid scratching with your nails.

Introducing your child to acupressure

Acupressure can be applied anywhere and any time, as
necessary. You can apply pressure directly on the skin or
through light clothing. Do not use oils or creams. Explain
exactly what you are doing and how it will help. Work

together to describe the kind of sensations that your child is feeling. Acupressure should never be painful.

Before you begin, both of you should take a few deep breaths to focus your attention on this time spent together.

Acupressure techniques

Over the years many different kinds of acupressure have been developed, each with different techniques, and they are used on the main acupressure points to balance the flow of Qi through the meridians. The simplest and most effective techniques for use with children are described below.

Pressure

One of the most commonly used techniques is applying stationary pressure for a length of time. Once you have located the point, apply pressure with the pads of your middle or index finger, or thumb. Pressure is usually applied in the direction of the flow of the meridian. Breathe out as you apply pressure, and in as you release the pressure.

Start with gentle pressure, then gradually increase it until your child feels a slight discomfort or sensitivity. Keep asking for feedback, and change your pressure if it becomes painful. Maintain a firm, steady, stationary pressure. You should start to feel the initial tenderness passing as the flow of Qi is balanced. Once the feeling passes, stop applying pressure. The length of time for which you hold the pressure will depend on how long your child is prepared to stay still, but aim for around 10 to 20 seconds. Do not continue with the treatment if your child feels unwell or faint.

Holding or stroking

This is a calming technique. Hold your thumb, finger or the palm of your hand over the acupressure point for a couple of minutes. Alternately, use a soothing, stroking action over the area.

Chronic or acute?

Chronic complaints are ongoing, such as hayfever or bedwetting. Acute complaints come on suddenly and are usually of limited duration such as tension headaches or travel sickness. For chronic complaints, work the points daily until the condition clears. For acute complaints, work them two or three times a day. Work on both sides of the body.

Ten common acupressure points

There are around 500 different points located along the meridians all over the body. Ten of the most common points are mentioned here. They are easy to locate and safe to use to help relieve common childhood ailments. Practise locating them on yourself first, then work together with your child to find where they lie on her body. Remember that the finger widths refer to those of the child being treated.

Depending on your child, you may choose to work the points to help with specific conditions, or select a few points to work daily or weekly as a preventative measure. This section is a guide to the location and benefits of the points. For suggestions on how to stimulate them to help ease a particular condition, turn to the relevant section in Chapter 5. Work on appropriate points on both sides of your child's body.

GV 20

Location: on the top of the head, directly above the tips of the ears and in line with the nose; you will feel a slight hollow, which may be a little sensitive to the touch.

Technique: apply pressure with the tip of one finger.

Benefits: calms fears and soothes nerves and irritability; boosts memory and concentration.

GV 24.5

Location: between the eyebrows at the top of the bridge of the nose and the lower edge of the forehead; feel for the slight indentation that is often known as the 'third eye point'.

Technique: use your first or second finger to apply pressure to this point; ask your child to tip her head slightly forward to increase the pressure – but ensure this feels comfortable.

Benefits: soothes feelings of irritability and confusion; eases headaches and stimulates the immune system; encourages clarity of vision and calms mind, body and spirit.

B 2

Location: just above the inner corner of each eye where the bridge of the nose meets the inner tip of the eyebrow; feel for two natural hollows, on either side of the nose.

Technique: press upwards with your thumbs or fingers, whichever feels most comfortable; work both points at the same time.

Benefits: relieves sinus pain, eye strain and headaches; eases the symptoms of hayfever.

SI 19

Location: in the slight depression in front of the ear; to locate it on yourself, first open your mouth a little way, then feel for the slight depression in front of the middle of your ear, close your mouth and your finger will be on the correct spot; invite your child to do the same.

Technique: use the pad of your index or middle fingers to apply pressure directed towards the ear.

Benefits: relieves earache; strengthens hearing and unblocks the ears after a flight.

GB 20

Location: on the bony ridge at the base of the skull. Trace the line along the bony ridge from the ears towards the centre. Feel for two slight hollows on either side of the neck between the two muscles.

Technique: rest the pads of your thumbs or fingers on these acupressure points, then ask your child to gently tilt her head back a little way, so that the weight of the head increases the pressure.

Benefits: relieves a stiff neck, tension headaches, colds, eye strain and insomnia.

P 6

Location: on the inside of the arm, about three finger widths above the natural crease on the wrist, between the two tendons.

Technique: support the wrist with your fingers and apply gentle pressure with the pad of your thumb. Repeat on the other forearm.

Benefits: relieves nausea, anxiety and travel sickness; eases wrist pain.

LI 4

Location: in the fleshy part between the thumb and fore-finger on the back of the hand.

Technique: place your forefinger underneath and your thumb on top; feel for the sensitive spot, then gently squeeze and hold. Repeat on the other hand.

Benefits: relieves constipation, indigestion, toothache, colds, sinusitis, shoulder pain and headaches; also useful for helping your child manage allergies.

H 7

Location: in the small hollow on the inner wrist, in line with the outer edge of the little finger.

Technique: apply gentle pressure with the pad of your thumb facing towards the little finger. Repeat on the other wrist.

Benefits: relieves insomnia; calms anxiety.

CV 6

Location: two finger widths directly below the belly button.

Technique: hold the palm of your hand or fingertips over this area, then press and hold for as long as feels comfortable, encouraging your child to breathe deeply. You can also rub or knead gently over this area.

Benefits: strengthens the lower back; boosts energy and vitality; stimulates the immune system and balances digestive disorders; useful for bedwetting and other urinary conditions.

St 36

Location: four finger widths below the kneecap, one finger width to the outside of the shinbone; to test that you are in the correct spot, try moving your child's foot up and down – you should feel a muscle flexing as you do this.

Technique: use the pad of your thumb or finger on this point. You can also rub this area briskly. Encourage your child to practise rubbing over the point on one leg with the heel of the opposite foot.

Benefits: strengthens the body; boosts the immune system; aids digestion; relieves nausea; eases knee pain.

Chapter 5: Treating common childhood ailments

Here are some easy-to-follow ways of embracing the healing power of touch to help your child overcome the minor symptoms of everyday ailments and prevent their recurrence. Different options are offered for each condition, so choose those that you and your child find most practical and effective. To locate the reflex areas and acupressure points, refer to Chapters 3 and 4. Do remember that although these natural remedies can be wonderfully beneficial, they are not a substitute for conventional medical advice and treatment.

Asthma

Recent research shows that children with asthma have benefited from regular reflexology sessions. While reflexology techniques are not appropriate during an acute attack, this simple routine can help ease anxiety and panic, open the airways and enable your child to breathe more freely during a mild attack. Use it on a regular weekly basis to help strengthen your child's respiratory system and support conventional medical care.

Reflexology sequence

1. Begin by pressing the pads of your thumbs on the solar plexus reflex points on both feet. This will help trigger the relaxation response. Hold for a count of three. Release the pressure. Repeat three times.

2. Now use your thumb to 'walk' or glide over the diaphragm line on the right foot, working from one side of the foot to the other. The diaphragm line follows the lower edge of the ball of the foot. Change hands and work back again.

3. Bring your thumb to the outer edge of the right big toe to work the throat and neck reflexes. Press, glide or 'walk' all around the base of the toe – underside, top and sides.

4. Use your thumb to 'walk' over the lung reflex area on the ball of the right foot. You can work in lines going upwards or across the foot, as you wish.

5. Gently press on the adrenal gland reflex point on the right foot with the pad of your thumb. Hold for a count of three. Release and repeat.

6. Repeat Steps 2–5 on the left foot.

Massage for asthma

Massage your child's back with generous sweeping movements in an upward direction. Massage through light clothing or use a small amount of plain carrier oil or Reassuring Back Rub.

Coughs and colds

On average a primary school child gets three to eight coughs and colds every year. Encourage your child to rest and drink plenty of fluids to boost her natural healing mechanisms. If she feels well enough for a massage, this soothing sequence – done in a sitting position – may ease some of the symptoms. If using oil, choose a small quantity of carrier oil or the Simple Massage and Bath Oil blend.

<u>Massage sequence</u>

1. Place your hands on your child's collar bones. Using the pads of your fingers, gently stroke outwards from the centre of the upper chest towards the arms. Release when you reach the arms and return to the starting position. Repeat this soothing stroke three or more times.

2. Now make small circular movements with the pads of your fingers, working outwards from the centre of the upper chest. Repeat.

3. Using the flat of your hands, gently pat over the upper chest area to help release any congestion and tightness.

4. Place one hand across your child's upper chest to offer reassurance. With the flat of the other hand, gently rub the back and up the neck, covering the whole area to help ease any aches and pains.

5. Starting on the right shoulder, stroke with the palm of one hand to midway down the back. Repeat with the other hand. As one hand finishes, the other begins,

in a wave-like movement. Cover the whole back with these stroking movements.

Reflexology for coughs and colds
Work the reflex areas for the neck and throat at the base of the big toes. Use your thumb to 'walk', glide or make small circular pressure movements around the base of the toe – underside, top and sides. Work the right foot followed by the left foot.

Sinus problems

Sinus problems are caused by inflammation of the membranes that line the nose. If your child suffers from ongoing sinus congestion, this gentle massage – performed in any position she finds comfortable and carried out without oils – can be most effective. Repeat two to three times daily. Your child may experience a 'popping' sensation in her head; reassure her that this is simply a sign that excess mucus is beginning to clear.

Massage sequence
1. Place your second or ring fingers in the small hollows on the inner edge of each of your child's eyebrows. Make three small circle movements, keeping your touch very gentle. Release. Move your fingers a little way along each eyebrow and repeat. Do the same on three more points. Check the pressure by asking for feedback.

2. Smooth over the eyebrows with the pads of two fingers, working from the inner to the outer corners. Continue the stroking movement over your child's temples towards her ears.

3. Place your fingers on either side of the bridge of your child's nose. Now stroke down the side of the nose with a comfortable pressure. Repeat.

4. Place the pads of your ring fingers in the slight hollow on the outside edges of the nostrils. Make three small circular movements.

5. Complete the sequence by stroking the pads of your fingers along the line of your child's cheekbones. Release when you reach the ears. Repeat three times.

Reflexology for sinus problems
Use your thumb and/or fingers to 'walk', glide or squeeze the sinus reflex areas on the back and side of each toe, starting at the base and working upwards. Work the right foot followed by the left foot.

Hayfever

Hayfever, an allergic reaction to pollen, is one of the most common allergic disorders in children over the age of five. When children are suffering from hayfever, they often find it hard to concentrate and their sleep may be disturbed. The causes and effects are different for everyone, so it is important to seek medical help. However, this reflexology sequence may help ease the symptoms and boost your child's immune system.

Reflexology routine
1. Start with your child's right foot. Support the foot with one hand, and use the thumb of your other hand to press

on the adrenal gland reflex. Hold for a count of three. Use a light touch on this area as it can be sensitive for some children.

2. Now work the head reflex area to help ease any fuzzy-headedness. With one hand keeping your child's big toe steady, use your other thumb to 'walk' or stroke over the whole of the padded area of the big toe.

3. Help to ease any congestion by working the sinus reflexes. Use your thumb and/or fingers to 'walk', glide or squeeze the back and sides of the big toe, starting at the base and working upwards. Repeat on each toe, repositioning your hands as necessary.

4. With the fingers of your supporting hand keeping the upper foot steady, use your working thumb to press on the eye reflex point located under the bend of the second toe. Hold for a count of three, or make three clockwise pressure movements.

5. Repeat Steps 1-4 on your child's left foot.

Acupressure for hayfever
Acupressure point B2 is useful for relieving the symptoms of hayfever and sinusitis. Hold and press in an upward direction for around 10–20 seconds, or as long as your child permits. Ask her to let her head fall slightly forwards onto your fingers, for maximum benefit. Use daily until the symptoms subside.

Tension headaches (Reflexology)

Most headaches in children are linked to stressful situations at school, at home or with friends. They usually start gradually and develop into a feeling of tightness in the head. Seek medical advice if they are recurrent, if the pain is severe or accompanied by fever, vomiting, a stiff neck or rash.

Reflexology sequence

1. Start with your child's right foot. Begin with the reflex associated with the main trouble-spot – the head. With one hand keeping the big toe steady, use your other thumb to 'walk' or stroke along it, covering the whole of the padded area of the big toe.

2. Now concentrate on calming the brain. Starting with the big toe, use your thumb to press on the top of it, just behind the nail. Hold for a count of three. Do the same on the next two toes. Keep the foot well supported with your other hand.

3. With one hand supporting the foot, use the thumb on your other hand to 'walk', glide or make small circular movements around the neck and throat reflex at the base of the big toe. Repeat.

4. Gently grasp your child's big toe and rotate it three times in one direction, then three times in the reverse direction.

5. Repeat Steps 1- 4 on your child's left foot

Cold compress for headaches

Encourage your child to lie down, then place a cool compress on her forehead. Use one drop each of lavender and

Roman chamomile to help relax any muscular tension and ease the pain.

Tension headaches (Massage)

Try this gentle tension-easing routine when your child has the first signs of a headache. Find a quiet place, dim the lighting and let fresh air circulate around the room. Keep your movements slow and controlled. It is intended to be done with your child in a sitting position, but can be adapted to lying down. If using oils, choose a small amount of carrier oil or the Simple Massage and Bath Oil blend.

<u>Massage sequence</u>

1. Begin by kneading your child's shoulders, because tension in this area often leads to headaches. With your fingers resting on her shoulders, use your thumbs to gently knead the soft muscle along the top of the shoulders. Press, lift, squeeze and release the flesh in a rhythmic, kneading action.

2. Now bring your hands to your child's temples, another tension hotspot. Using the pads of two fingers, massage the temples with small circular movements. Avoid digging in with your fingers. Keep your fingers on the same spot – it is the skin that moves as you make the rotations.

3. Place the palms of your hands on your child's forehead. Stroke upwards from the eyebrows to the hairline, with one hand following the other in a wave-like movement. Cover the whole forehead.

4. With your hands in a claw-like position, rest them on your child's scalp. Use the fleshy pads of your fingers and thumbs to make small circular movements, 'shampooing' all over the scalp. Continue as long as you wish.

5. Finish the routine by resting your hands on your child's head. Hold for as long as feels comfortable to her.

Acupressure for headaches
Use acupressure point GB 20 to ease tension in the neck and head. Rest the pads of your thumbs or fingers here. Now ask your child to tilt her head back a little, to increase the pressure. Hold for 20–30 seconds, or as long as feels comfortable.

Eye strain

Working at a computer screen or watching television can put a strain on the muscles in the eyes. Do ensure that your child's eyes are examined regularly to check for any visual problems that may need correcting. If your child complains of tired eyes, use this simple massage sequence – carried out in any position, without oils – to relieve the strain and clear her vision.

Massage sequence
1. Rub the palms of your hands together so that they feel warm.

2. Cup your palms over her eyes, closing your fingers to cut out as much light as possible. This 'palming' technique is useful for self-help. It is particularly restful for the eyes to be in total darkness.

3. Bring your palms to your child's cheeks and stroke towards the ears in a gentle smoothing action to help boost the blood circulation to this area. Repeat several times.

4. Next, tap around the eye area using the pads of your fingers of both hands in a gentle action. Maintain a light pressure and avoid working directly over the eyes.

5. Gently stroke your child's forehead, including the eyebrows, using the palms of your hands. Stroke across the forehead from the centre outwards, with both hands working at the same time. Keep the movement soft and flowing. Finish the sequence by repeating the 'palming' action.

Reflexology for eye strain
Work the eye reflex area on both feet, starting with the right foot. With the fingers of your supporting hand keeping your child's foot steady, use your working thumb to press on the reflex point located on the ball of the foot, under the first bend of the second toe. Hold for a count of three, or make three clockwise pressure movements.

Sleep problems (Massage)

A regular bedtime massage can soothe your child, mentally and physically, encouraging a peaceful night's sleep. Set time aside – after a warm bath is ideal – so that the experience is calm for you both. Keep your strokes gentle, slow and rhythmic, with lots of repetition so that your child feels safe and nurtured. Begin with her lying on her front or side; this massage is best carried out without oils, over nightwear.

Massage sequence

1. Place both hands on your child's upper back, then trail one hand down the back with a long, feather-like stroke. When one hand reaches the lower back, the other one begins another stroke. Continue this rhythmic pattern with alternate hands stroking in one flowing move.

2. Ask your child to roll over on her back. Bring your hands to her head and trace small, slow circular movements over her scalp with the pads of your thumbs and fingers. Massage all areas of her scalp that you can comfortably reach.

3. Continue these small circles over her forehead, temples and cheeks using the pads of your fingers. Keep your touch very light and slow.

4. Cover her forehead in gentle, reassuring strokes, working in a downward direction. You may find this more comfortable with the backs of your hands. As one stroke finishes, so the next begins.

5. Place your hands on your child's head, fingertips just touching. Gently cup the head and let the warmth of your hands comfort her into sleepy relaxation.

Acupressure for sleep problems

Acupressure point H7 is helpful when your child wakes frequently at night. Apply gentle pressure, with the pad of your thumb facing towards the little finger. Release and repeat on the other wrist.

Sleep problems (Reflexology)

If your child is restless at night and you are quite sure she is not unwell, then this gentle reflexology sequence may help her to settle down. This simple routine can be very effective in slowing the breath, quietening any anxieties and clearing the mind in preparation for sound sleep.

Reflexology sequence

1. Begin with some diaphragm rocking. Place your thumb on the diaphragm line on the outside edge of the right foot. As you gently press in, use your other hand to rock the toes forward. Release the pressure and gently rock them back. Repeat until your thumb reaches the inner edge of the diaphragm line. Change hands and repeat on the left foot.

2. Now enjoy some solar plexus soothing. Place the pad of your thumbs on the solar plexus reflex points on your child's feet to help calm and relax her whole system. Gently press and hold for a count of three. Release your pressure. Repeat three times.

3. Still grasping both your child's feet with your hands, bring your thumbs to the big toes and make small circular pressures over the head and brain reflex areas on the fleshy pads and top of the big toe and on the tops of the next two toes.

4. Finish by cradling your child's heels in the palms of your hands. Hold for a few minutes. This comforting hold feels just like the kind of 'hug' your child needs to drift off to sleep.

Scented pillow for sleep problems

Place one drop only of lavender essential oil on the corner of the underside of your child's pillow or on the collar or back of her pyjamas. This enables the sleep-inducing aroma of lavender to float around the room, without running the risk of getting any essential oil in your child's eyes.

Bedwetting

Bedwetting can affect young children, especially when they are very tired or anxious. As bladder function matures, most children start to gain control at night, but if you have any concerns, or your child complains of pain when passing urine, seek medical advice. Waking up in a wet bed can shake a child's confidence. A gentle reflexology session at bedtime offers you the opportunity to support your child with a positive, caring attitude.

Reflexology sequence

1. Begin by gently stroking down the instep of your child's right foot with the palms of your hands. Keep the movements slow and nurturing. Repeat on the left foot. Use these stroking movements at intervals during your reflexology session.

2. Now work on the right foot. With the foot well supported, use your thumb to 'walk' or glide over the bladder reflex area several times. If the area is not well defined, walk or glide across the middle of the sole of the foot.

3. Move to the adrenal gland reflex area. Support the foot with one hand and gently press on this reflex point with the pad of your other thumb. Hold for a count of three, using a light touch.

4. Still supporting the foot with one hand, use your other thumb to 'walk' or glide along the spine reflex area on the inner edge of the foot. Work in one direction, then change hands and work back in the other direction.

5. Use your thumb to 'walk' or glide over the diaphragm reflex area, working from one side of the foot to the other. The diaphragm line is located along the lower edge of the ball of the foot. Change hands and work back again.

6. Repeat Steps 2–5 on the left foot.

Acupressure for bedwetting
Acupressure point CV 6 can be helpful for bedwetting. Hold the palm of your hand or fingertips over this area. Press for as long as feels comfortable. Encourage your child to breathe deeply. You can also stroke this area gently or hold it with loving care.

Tummy ache

Tummy ache is very common in childhood. There are many physical causes, but it can also be a way of expressing anxiety. If you are worried, seek medical advice. However, this simple massage – carried out with your child lying on her back – can offer reassurance to talk through her concerns. Use very gentle pressure as the stomach may feel delicate. If using oil, choose a small amount of carrier oil or Tummy Soothing Oil.

<u>Massage sequence</u>

1. Place the palm of one hand on your child's tummy. Now place your other palm on top. Use a gentle pressure that is comfortable for your child.

2. Make a few small circles around her tummy-button area, with your hands stroking in a clockwise direction. Gradually increase the size of these comforting circles so that they cover the whole of the tummy area. Do around 20 circles. Keep the pressure comfortable for your child.

3. Now place one palm just below the ribs. Stroke the whole palm to the bottom of the tummy, using a gentle, even pressure. When one hand finishes a stroke, the other hands begins. Continue to use alternate hands in a wave-like movement for around 20 strokes.

4. Finish by holding both of your palms on the tummy. The heat generated by them will have a relaxing effect on your child's whole body.

Aromatic bath for tummy ache

Suggest that your child soaks in an aromatic bath to help calm her tummy and relax her mind. Fill the bath with water, then add a small quantity of Calming Bath blend and agitate the water. This can be especially helpful if tummy aches are preventing your child getting to sleep.

Constipation

Mild constipation is a fairly common childhood complaint and usually lasts only a few days. However, sluggish bowel movements or difficulty in passing stools can be distressing for your child. A daily reflexology session can ease discomfort and stimulate bowel function. Encourage your child to take regular exercise and to drink plenty of water to maintain regular bowel movements. Start the routine by using some of the relaxation techniques described in Chapter 3.

Reflexology sequence

1. After relaxing both feet, work the liver and gall bladder reflexes, which are found mainly on the right foot. Use your thumb to 'walk' or glide over the area, starting from the outside edge of the foot. Change hands and work in the opposite direction.

2. Now work the small and large intestine reflex areas on the right foot. Support your child's foot with one hand and use the thumb on your other hand to 'walk' or glide over the area, working from the outside edge of the foot across to the inner edge.

3. Work the small and large intestine reflex areas on the left foot. Support your child's foot with one hand and use the thumb on your other hand to 'walk' or glide over the area, working from the outside edge of the foot across to the inner edge.

4. Work the adrenal gland reflex by using the pad of your thumb to press on this area on your child's right foot. Hold for a count of three. Do the same on your child's left foot.

5. Finish with some solar plexus soothing. With your hands supporting the sides of each foot, hold your thumbs on the solar plexus points. Ask your child to breathe in as you press on them and breathe out as you release the pressure. Repeat three times.

Acupressure for constipation
Acupressure point LI 4 can help relieve constipation and accompanying headaches. Place your forefinger beneath it and your thumb on top. Gently squeeze and hold for 20–30 seconds, or as long as feels comfortable to your child. Release and repeat on the other hand.

Travel sickness
When a child suffers from travel sickness, long journeys by road, sea or air are usually miserable for everyone. The symptoms are linked to disturbances of the inner ear and are often made worse by anxiety. Try using this reflexology sequence before travelling to help balance the inner ear and calm your child. Ginger and peppermint (taken as a biscuit, sweet or drink) can also be settling for the stomach. If travelling by car, keep it well ventilated.

Reflexology sequence
1. Start by working on your child's right foot. Press on the adrenal gland reflex to help calm the body. Hold for a count of three.

2. With the foot well supported, press on the ear reflex point, located on the ball of the foot under the first bend of the little toe. Hold for a count of three or

70

make three circular pressure movements in a clockwise direction.

3. Now work the neck reflex area. With one hand supporting the foot, use your other thumb to 'walk' or glide all around the base of the big toe. Repeat.

4. Finish by working the diaphragm reflex. Use your thumb to 'walk' or glide along the line, from one side of the foot to the other and back again.

5. Repeat Steps 1- 4 on your child's left foot.

Acupressure for travel sickness
Acupressure point HP 6 (the point used by anti-sickness wristbands) is helpful for calming the queasiness associated with movement. Measure three finger widths – using your child's fingers – from the crease of your child's wrist. Now apply pressure with the pad of your thumb. Hold for around 20–30 seconds. Release and repeat on the other arm.

Earache

Earache is often linked to an infection following a cold or tonsillitis, although there are many other causes. Seek immediate medical advice if earache is combined with high temperature, fever, swelling around the ear, drowsiness, vomiting, loss of balance or hearing, discharge from the ear, a neck pain or rash, or if you feel concerned. This reflexology routine is designed to target the main reflex areas linked with earache and will complement conventional medical treatment.

Reflexology sequence

1. Start with your child's right foot. With the fingers of your supporting hand keeping the upper foot steady, use your working thumb to press on the ear reflex point under first bend of the little toe. Hold for a count of three, or make three circular pressure movements in a clockwise direction.

2. Repeat this movement on the eye reflex point, located under the first bend of the second toe.

3. Now work on the sinus reflex area. Depending on the size of your child's toes, use your thumb or fingers to 'walk', glide or squeeze the back and sides of the big toe, starting at the base and working upwards. Repeat on each toe in turn, repositioning your hands as necessary.

4. Finish the routine by working the adrenal gland reflex area. Press on the point with your thumb. Hold and then release.

5. Repeat Steps 1- 4 on your child's left foot.

Acupressure for earache

Acupressure point SI 19 can help to relieve earache and unblock ears after a flight. Locate it on yourself, and ask your child to do the same. Use the pad of your index or middle fingers to apply pressure towards the ear. Hold for around 10–20 seconds or as long as feels comfortable to your child.

Eczema

Eczema is an itchy red rash that can develop anywhere on the body and is linked with an allergy to foods or environmental factors. Stress and anxiety can also be triggers. It is highly irritating for children, who naturally want to scratch their skin, which can lead to infection. It is important to keep the skin moist and supple, avoiding fissures that can result in complications. Use a light moisturizing cream or oil for this calming reflexology sequence.

Reflexology sequence

1. Support your child's right foot with your left hand. Use your thumb to 'walk' or glide over the liver and gall bladder reflex area found mainly on the right foot. Start from the outer edge of the foot and work inwards. Change hands and work in the opposite direction.

2. Now work the small and large intestine areas on your child's right foot to help cleanse the system. Use your thumb to 'walk' or glide over the area, working from the outside edge of the foot across to the inner edge.

3. Work the small and large intestine areas on your child's left foot. Use your thumb to 'walk' or glide over the area, working from the outside edge of the foot across to the inner edge. Keep the foot well supported.

4. Still supporting the left foot, work the spleen reflex, which is located only on the left foot. Use your thumb to 'walk' or glide over the area.

5. Finish with some diaphragm rocking which is often a favourite with children. Place your thumb on the diaphragm line on the outside edge of the right foot. As you gently press in, use your other hand to rock the toes forward. Release and rock them back. Repeat until your thumb reaches the inner edge of the diaphragm line. Repeat on the left foot.

Moisturizing bath for eczema

Soothe mild eczema irritation with a cool, moisturizing bath. Add 10 ml sweet almond oil or coconut oil to the water and gently agitate it. While your child is soaking in the bath or drying herself afterwards, encourage her to rub oil into her skin. Do wash the bath afterwards so it is not slippery.

Tense neck and shoulders

Poor posture leads to shoulder and neck tension, which can give rise to stiffness, poor circulation, headaches and eye strain. This massage sequence – carried out with your child in a sitting position – can help relax tense muscles and encourage healthy circulation. Aim to massage your child daily if she is studying hard for exams. If using oil, choose a small amount of carrier oil or the Reassuring Back Rub.

Massage sequence

1. Place your hands on your child's upper back, one on either side of the spine. With your fingers pointing upward, stroke your hands up and around the shoulder blades, tracing generous circles. Keep the movement

slow and smooth, with more pressure on the upward movement. Repeat three times.

2. With your hands resting on the shoulders, gently knead the soft flesh beneath between your palms and fingers. Press, lift, squeeze and release. Do not press too hard or too suddenly. Then gently stroke the area.

3. Support your child's forehead with one hand. With the flat of two or three fingers of the other hand, rub lightly and briskly around the back of the neck and under the base of the skull.

4. Bring your hands to the base of the neck and stroke along the top of the shoulders and down to the elbows. Release the pressure and glide back to the starting position. Repeat three times.

5. Finish the routine by resting your hands, palms downward, on your child's shoulders. Hold for a count of three. Ask your child to take three deep breaths, in and out.

Reflexology for a tense neck
With one hand supporting your child's toes, use your other thumb to 'walk' or glide around the neck reflexes located around the base of the big toe on each foot.

Growing pains

Pains associated with growth can sometimes occur in childhood, especially those aged seven to twelve. The soreness is usually in the limbs and may cause a child to wake at night feeling disorientated. Massaging the area with love is just what your child needs. Before massaging, check there are no injuries that could be the underlying cause.

<u>Massage sequence</u>
1. Place your hands over the affected area. Hold it, letting the warmth of your hands offer comfort and ease the aches and pains.

2. Gently stroke over the whole area with the palms of your hands moving in an upward direction, one hand following the other in a wave-like motion. Repeat several times.

3. Repeat the same action, this time making small circular movements, with the palms of your hands moving in an upward direction.

4. Finish by holding your hands over the affected area. If possible, stay with your child for as long as she needs you, in order to find reassurance and feel the pain ease.

Comforting bath for growing pains
Invite your child to lie in a warm bath infused with essential oils to ease her growing aches and pains. Fill the bath with water, then add a small quantity of the Comforting Bath blend and gently agitate the water.

Stress (Reflexology)

All children react differently to stressful situations, and it may not always be easy to identify when a child is finding it hard to cope. Touch therapy can help counterbalance the detrimental effects of stress and boost your child's self-esteem. Experiencing positive relaxation from a young age will help your child cope with stress in later life. Use this reflexology sequence to enjoy a peaceful time together, away from the demands of everyday life.

Reflexology sequence

1. Cradle your child's heels in the palms of your hands. Hold for a few seconds to offer reassurance.

2. Sandwich your child's right foot between your palms. Keeping your hands soft, move the flat of your hands gently backward and forward across the top and bottom of the foot to create a rocking sensation. Repeat on the left foot.

3. Help your child to relax with some gentle diaphragm rocking. Place your thumb on the diaphragm line on the outside edge of the right foot. As you gently press in, use your other hand to rock the toes forward. Release and gently rock them back. Repeat until your thumb reaches the inner edge of the diaphragm line. Repeat on the left foot.

4. Next work on the adrenal gland reflex to counterbalance the effects of stress. Use your thumb to press lightly on this reflex on your child's right foot. Repeat on the left foot.

5. Finish with some solar plexus soothing. With your hands supporting the sides of each foot, hold your thumbs on

the solar plexus points for a count of three. Ask your child to breathe in as you press on them and breathe out as you release the pressure. Repeat three times.

Foot bath for stress
Offer your child a soothing footbath using the Relaxing Foot Mix. Suggest that she lets the warmth and aroma of the footbath help her relax while talking to you, reading a book or listening to some gentle music.

Stress (Massage)

When your child appears overwhelmed with the stresses of life, suggest offering her a gentle massage. She will start to relax under your caring touch and may be more willing to share her worries. This routine is intended to be done with your child in a sitting position, but can be adapted to lying down. If using oils, choose a small amount of carrier oil or the Simple Massage and Bath Oil blend.

Massage sequence
1. Rest your hands, palms downward, on your child's head. Hold for a count of three. Children often find it hard to 'let go' of their concerns, so invite her to put all her stresses into an imaginary balloon or bubble and then release it and imagine watching it floating far, far away.

2. Now stroke both hands from the top of her head downwards, over her shoulders and upper back in a long, sweeping movement. Release. Bring your hands back to the top of the head and repeat this soothing stroke. Ask whether she likes the movement to cover her ears or fall behind them.

3. Starting on the right shoulder, stroke with the palm of one hand to midway down the back. Repeat with the other hand. As one hand finishes, the other begins. Work across the back with this wave-like movement.

4. Place the heels of your hands over your child's temples, with your fingers facing away from you. Make slow, circular movements over the area. Repeat three to four times.

5. Gently stroke your child's forehead using the palms of your hands. Stroke upward or across the forehead from one side to the other. Keep the movements soft and flowing.

Aromatic tissue for stress
Place one drop of lavender, mandarin or Roman chamomile essential oil on a paper tissue or cotton handkerchief. Wrap in cling film and invite your child to keep it in his pocket to sniff when he needs it.

Anxiety

Anxiety can be triggered by many factors and can manifest in various ways, sometimes making a child physically unwell. If there is no apparent or medical reason, this breathing sequence followed by an arm and hand massage may help calm the child. She can sit or lie in a comfortable position, with her hands by her sides. If using oil, choose a small amount of carrier oil or the Simple Massage and Bath Oil blend.

Massage sequence
1. Follow this breathing exercise together. Breathe in deeply through the nose. Imagine the abdomen is

filling with air, like a balloon. Slowly release the air until the abdomen feels empty, pushing it out with a hissing noise. It may help if your child rests one hand on her abdomen to get used to the feel. Repeat twice more.

2. Begin the massage with your child's right hand. Hold it, palm downward, between your own palms. Enjoy a few moments of stillness and comforting warmth. Release your hold very gradually by sliding your hands towards the fingertips and then gently and slowly drawing away.

3. Now hold your child's right arm between your hands and gently squeeze, release and hold. Move your hands further up the arm and repeat. Work right up to the shoulders and back down to the wrist.

4. Supporting the wrist with one hand, stroke your other palm all the way up the arm from the wrist to the shoulder. Release and glide gently back to the starting position. This is wonderfully reassuring. Repeat as often as you wish.

5. With your child's hand facing downward, place one hand beneath it for support. Gently stroke the hand, letting the strokes get progressively lighter and slower.

6. Repeat Steps 2- 5 on the left arm.

Reflexology for anxiety
Try some solar plexus soothing which helps to relax mind and body. Press the pads of your thumbs on the

solar plexus points on both feet and hold for a count of three. Repeat three times. Ask your child to breathe in as you press in and breathe out as you release the pressure.

Fears and phobias

Snakes, monsters, strangers, darkness...Young children tend to experience more fears and phobias than adults and often feel the emotion far more intensely. In some instances medical help may be necessary, but most intense fears are a natural part of growing up and can be conquered with support, listening and understanding. This relaxing reflexology routine offers your child the opportunity for some individual attention and reassurance.

Reflexology sequence
1. Cradle your child's heels in the palms of your hands. Hold for a few seconds. This feels like a reassuring hug. Then slowly slide your hands away.

2. Continue to offer relaxation and reassurance by working on the solar plexus points on both feet. Press the pads of your thumbs on the points on both feet. Hold for a count of three. Release the pressure and repeat three times.

3. With your child's right foot well supported, use your thumb to 'walk' or glide down the edge of the foot, starting at the big toe. This is the spine reflex area. Move in a forward direction, following the foot's natural curve. Change hands and 'walk' or glide back up to the big toe.

4. Use the thumb of your other hand to press on the brain reflex on top of the big toe, just behind the nail. Hold for a count of three. Do the same on the next two toes.

5. Repeat Steps 3 and 4 on your child's left foot.

Acupressure for fears and phobias

Acupressure point GV 24.5 is useful for calming mind, body and spirit. Feel for the slight indentation between the eyebrows at the top of the bridge of the nose. Apply pressure on this point or gently stroke the area for around 10–20 seconds.

Hyperactivity

Some children seem to be constantly 'on the go', unwilling to sit still for any length of time. This can be draining for parents, and can lead to tension within the whole family. If at first your child will not cooperate with this reflexology routine, keep trying – even if only for a few minutes. A hyperactive child may soon benefit from experiencing how good it feels to be calm and relaxed, with your full attention.

Reflexology sequence

1 Start with a simple foot massage to help calm your child. With your hands cradling her right foot, gently massage the soles of the foot with the fleshy pads of your thumbs. Move your thumbs in circles using a gentle, even pressure, covering the whole of the sole. Repeat on the left foot.

2. Continue to help calm your child with solar plexus soothing. Press the pads of your thumbs on the points

on both feet. Suggest that your child takes a deep, relaxing breath in as you press on the points. Release your pressure and ask her to take a breath out. Repeat three times.

3. Now work on the brain reflex area on the right foot. Starting with the big toe, press your thumb on the top of the toe, just behind the nail. Hold for a count of three. Do the same on the next two toes. Repeat on the left foot.

4. Move to the adrenal gland reflex point on the right foot. Use your thumb to press and hold for a count of three. Use a light touch as this area can be sensitive, especially if your child is experiencing a lot of stress. Repeat on the left foot.

Aromatic bath for hyperactivity
Soothe your child with an aromatic bath. Run the bath as usual, then add around 5 ml of Calming Bath mix. Agitate the water, then follow your usual bathtime routine.

Fatigue

It is perfectly normal for children to get tired, especially if they have a hectic schedule. However, if you are concerned that your child seems persistently tired, seek medical advice. The best way to prevent tiredness is to ensure your child has a healthy lifestyle with plenty of nourishing food, regular exercise and sleep. This stimulating massage sequence – carried out with your child in a sitting position, without the use of oils – can also be the perfect pick-me-up.

Massage sequence

1. With one hand resting on your child's left shoulder, place your other hand on your child's right shoulder. Using the palm of your hand, make generous sweeping strokes across the top of the left shoulder and around the shoulder blade. Repeat three times. Change hands and massage the other right side.

2. Place one hand across your child's upper chest to offer support. With the flat of the other hand, rub across the upper back, tops of the shoulders and upper arms in small zigzag, energizing movements. Rub briskly, covering the whole area.

3. Using the flat of your hands, gently pat from the top of the right shoulder all the way down the arm to your child's hands and back up again. Repeat several times. Your hands work alternately. Repeat in the left arm.

4. Rest your hands lightly on your child's head. Using your fingers, gently rub over the scalp, working from the front of the head to the back. Check that the pressure feels comfortable.

5. Now gently drum the pads of your fingers in a random fashion all over your child's head. Continue this light, bouncy tabla movement over the shoulders and neck.

Acupressure for fatigue

Acupressure point St 36 is useful for combating lethargy. Use the pad of your thumb or finger on this point, with pressure directed towards the knee. Hold for 20–30 seconds or as long as feels comfortable, release and repeat, or rub briskly for 30 seconds.

Exam nerves

Children face the pressure of exams from a young age. Offer them nourishing meals and plenty of fluids, and encourage them to take regular exercise to rid the body of stress hormones. This supportive massage can help ease nerves and offer reassurance. If using oil, choose a small amount of carrier oil or Reassuring Back Rub.

Massage sequence

1. Stand behind your child. With your hands resting on your child's shoulders, ask her to raise her shoulders as she breathes in, then release them as she breathes out with a large sigh. She will start to feel the tension dissipating. Repeat three times.

2. Now gently knead the soft flesh on the top of her shoulders with your palms and fingers. Press, lift, squeeze and release in a rhythmic action, like kneading bread dough. Be careful not to press too hard or too suddenly. Then gently stroke the area.

3. With your hands on the top of the right arm, gently squeeze, release and hold. Move your hands further down the arm and repeat. Work down to the elbow and back up to the top of the arm. Repeat on the left arm.

4. Bring your hands to the base of your child's neck, your right hand on right side of the neck, and your

left hand on the left. Stroke along the shoulders and down the arms to the elbow. Release the pressure and glide gently back. Repeat three times.

5. Finish by placing your index and second finger over your child's temples, with your fingers facing away from you. Your right hand is on the right temple, and your left hand on the left temple. Make slow, circular movements. Repeat three to four times. This is also a very effective self-help technique to teach your child.

Breathing exercises for exam nerves
Try some gentle breathing exercises with your child. Ask your child to take three deep breaths, in and out. Ask her to imagine that she is breathing in peace and calm and breathing out her worries about the exam. Repeat three times.

Chapter 6: Self-help tool kit

Children who grow up enjoying the benefits of nurturing touch in the family home learn to recognize the importance of looking after their own health and well-being. Share these simple self-help tips with your child to introduce her to ways of alleviating minor symptoms with her own natural healing resources. You may find them helpful for yourself too.

Anxiety

Teach your child how to use this simple routine to overcome feelings of anxiety and restore his sense of control over a stressful situation. The movements can be so discreet that no one need know just how your child is managing to stay so calm and focused. Encourage him to practise the sequence every day until it becomes second nature to him.

Reflexology sequence
1. Grip your right thumb between the palm and fingers of your left hand. Squeeze gently. Hold until you feel a pulse. Release. Move to your next finger and again

squeeze gently until you feel a pulse. Repeat with all the fingers on your right hand.

2. Now repeat Step 1 on your left hand.

3. Place your right thumb in the centre of your left palm. This is your solar plexus point. As you apply pressure to this point, take a deep breath in. Exhale and release the pressure. Repeat at least three times. As you slowly breathe in, imagine that you are taking in feelings of calmness and peace. As you breathe out, try to release any tensions and anxieties.

4. Change hands and repeat Step 3 on the other hand. This simple exercise helps calm and relax the whole nervous system. It is one of the most popular self-help techniques for children and adults of all ages.

Massage for anxiety
Massage your solar plexus, a meeting point for a network of nerves that is located just below your breastbone in line with your chin. With the pads of your fingers on one hand, use gentle pressure to make ten small anti-clockwise circles over your solar plexus. Now hold your solar plexus. Focus on letting your breathing become slow and controlled.

Tummy tension
Children can experience tummy aches and pains for many different reasons. If you are sure there is no underlying medical cause, then encourage your child to use this soothing sequence when her tummy feels out of balance.

The series of moves, which can be carried out sitting or lying down, also helps ease period pains and premenstrual tummy cramps for older girls. Suggest that she keeps the pressure light, with plenty of comforting repetitions.

Massage sequence
1. Place your left hand on the top half of your tummy. Use the flat of your right hand to trace ten gentle circles around your navel.

2. Now place the flat of both hands on your tummy, with your fingers pointing downwards. Bring your hands up and then away from each other, in an outward circular movement. Your hands meet again at the bottom and continue to form two separate circles. Repeat as often as you wish.

3. Trace the same path with your hands as in Step 2, this time making light circular moves with the pads of your fingertips.

4. Stroke the whole area with very light pressure. Your hands should move slowly and gently in an upward direction, working alternately or at the same time, whichever feels most comforting.

Herbal tea for tummy tension
Cut back on stimulating drinks such as cola and try herbal teas instead. Peppermint, ginger and chamomile teas are all helpful for easing stomach pains and cramps.

Concentration

Most children find that their attention starts to wander from time to time – especially during homework and revision. Show your child this massage sequence when his level of concentration begins to dip. If your child needs an instant pep-up in a short space of time, suggest that he chooses just one or two of these moves.

<u>Massage sequence</u>

1. Place your right hand on top of your left shoulder. Knead the fleshy area here between your fingers and the heel of your hand. Continue for as long as feels good. Repeat with your left hand on your right shoulder. Enjoy the feeling of tension release. Try leaning on a table to do this move if it feels easier.

2. With the flat of your right hand, rub briskly across the top of your left shoulder and all the way down the arm to your hand. Repeat this stimulating move with your left hand on your right arm.

3. Now use the flat of both hands to pat gently all over your head, neck and face. Your hands can move simultaneously or alternately, whichever feels best. Continue in a random fashion for as long as you wish.

4. Place your hands on top of your head and stroke down over your neck and the top of your shoulders. Again, your hands can move at the same time or one after the other. Repeat several times.

5. Finish the sequence by shaking both hands loosely from the wrists.

Acupressure for concentration
Acupressure point GV 20 is useful for boosting memory and concentration. You will feel a slight hollow on top of the head directly above with the tips of the ears, and in line with the nose, which may be a little sensitive. Press and hold until you feel any tenderness easing.

Stressed hands

Mobile phones, computers, electronic games ... In our modern technological world, children's hands are required to carry out many repetitive moves and can easily become over-worked and painful. Encourage your child to do this gentle stretching and massage routine several times during the day when she is placing heavy demands on her hands. Do advise her to stop or limit her movements if she experiences any pain or discomfort.

Massage sequence
1. Make soft fists with both hands. Then splay your fingers and thumbs, giving them a gentle stretch. Hold for a count of five. Release and repeat.

2. Grasp your right thumb between the forefingers and thumb of your left hand. Hold. Now pull gently, to give the whole thumb a stretch. Slide your hand to the top of the thumb, then let your fingers float away from the tip.

3. Repeat Step 2 on all fingers of your right hand.

4. Clasp your right hand in your left hand, and use your left thumb to knead your right palm with small circular rotations. Work all over the palm, especially the muscular pad at the base of the thumb.

5. Repeat the whole sequence on your left hand.

Aromatic hand therapy
Bathe your hands in a bowl half-full of warm water. Add a small quantity of Relaxing Hand Mix, gently agitate the water and then let your hands enjoy a soothing soak for around three to five minutes.

Headache

Tension headaches respond well to gentle massage. Show your child how to use these simple moves to help relax the muscles of the head, neck and face, thereby boosting the circulation and relieving the pain. Encourage your child to use this sequence at the first signs of a headache. She can experiment with different levels of pressure to discover what feels most effective without making the symptoms worse.

Massage sequence
1. Cradle your head in your hands, with your fingers meeting at the top of your head. As you breathe out, exert gentle pressure with your hands. As you breathe in, release the pressure. Move your hands a little further back and repeat.

2. Place one hand on top of your head. Gently knead your scalp between your fingers and the heel of your hand.

Cover the whole of your scalp with this relaxing move. Repeat with the other hand.

3. Tilt your head forward a little. Support your forehead with one hand, and use the palm of your other hand to stroke the back of your neck gently in a large circular movement. Repeat several times.

4. Place both hands on your head, thumbs resting on the bony ridge at the back. Make small circular movements with your thumbs along the ridge, from the centre towards your ears. Release. Return to the start and repeat.

5. Finish the sequence with some slow, nurturing strokes across your forehead. Stroke for as long as you wish.

Reflexology for headaches
Work on the head and brain reflex areas on your hands. Use your right thumb to 'walk' or stoke over the top of your left thumb, and the whole of the padded area. Repeat on the right thumb.

Toothache

When toothache strikes, the pain can be almost unbearable. The first course of action is to contact your child's dentist, who will be able to identify the cause and suggest a treatment plan. In the meantime, encourage your child to try this easy-to-follow hand reflexology sequence, to help ease the pain. It works the reflexes to the face and teeth, which are located on the back of the thumbs and the next two fingers.

Reflexology routine

1. Grasp your right thumb between the first two fingers and thumb of your left hand. Use your left thumb to 'walk' or stroke across the back of the right thumb. Start just below the nail and work in lines towards the wrist.

2. Do the same movement on the index and second fingers of your right hand.

3. Now use your left thumb to press just beneath the nail of the right thumb. Use a pressure that feels comfortable. Hold for a count of five. Release and repeat.

4. Repeat this press-and-hold action on the index and second fingers.

5. Repeat the whole sequence on the left hand.

Acupressure for toothache

Acupressure point LI 4 is effective for toothache. Place your forefinger beneath the fleshy part on the hand between thumb and forefinger, and your thumb on top. Feel for the sensitive spot. Gently squeeze and hold. Repeat on the other hand. *Do not use during pregnancy.*

Leg cramp

Cramp in calf muscles is quite common in children, especially those actively involved in exercise. Although it does not usually last longer than 15 minutes, it can be very painful – and often happens when least expected. So encourage your child to learn this simple stretch-and-massage routine to help relieve the spasm and prevent it recurring. If possible, elevate the affected leg to aid healthy circulation of blood to the calf muscles.

<u>Massage sequence</u>

1. Sit with your legs outstretched in front of you. Place the foot of the affected leg on top of the other foot. Pull your toes gently towards you. Hold for as long as feels comfortable. Release. Repeat until you feel a gradual easing of the cramping sensation.

2. Now gently knead, squeeze and roll your calf muscle between your fingers and thumb and the palm of your hand. This helps to boost the blood's circulation and ease any tension in the muscle, to prevent further cramping.

3. Finish by stroking from your ankles to your knees, with one hand following the other, to soothe the whole area.

Preventing cramp

Prevent cramp by making a real effort to warm up properly before doing lots of exercise. Cramp is often linked to dehydration, so drinking water before, during and after exercise or playing sport may also be beneficial.

Acknowledgements

Firstly, love and thanks to our two wonderful daughters, Lizi and Emma, with whom I have shared the many benefits of positive touch over the years.

This book has been greeted with enormous enthusiasm from the very first discussions right through to publication so my thanks to my ever-supportive agents, Chelsey Fox and Charlotte Howard. Practical help and constructive advice on content came from many people especially my friends and therapists: Takiko Ando, Sandra Hooper, Lynne Booth, Anne Bennett, Kristine Walker, Ronni Pettifer and Toni Mcgloin.

I am very grateful to Carolyn Story, Chief Executive of the Association of Reflexologists (AoR), and members of the AoR team, especially Laura Franzen and Sally Earlam, for their support of the book and provision of foot maps.

The popularity of this book in its first edition was one of the inspirations for the founding of the successful Story Massage project. For more information on Story Massage for Children please visit: www.storymassage.co.uk

Picture Acknowledgements

Association of Reflexologists (Foot Maps)
Kristine Walker (The 10 Zones of the body, Caterpillar walk)

About the author

Mary Atkinson is an award-winning complementary therapy practitioner and tutor. She has her own training school running accredited courses for therapists and beginners wishing to share the benefits of touch therapies with others. She is author of over 15 books including *The Art of Indian Head Massage* and *Once Upon A Touch ... Story Massage for Children*. She lives in Chichester with her husband and has two grown-up daughters.

Printed in Great Britain
by Amazon